Clinical Cases in Dermatologic Surgery

T0357916

Acknowledgments

We have learned a great deal through our joint collaboration and also from our truly outstanding contributing authors. We would like to thank them all most sincerely for their excellent work and the intellectual stimulation they provided. In many cases, we have been delighted to discover a new approach or modification to the common problems we cover in this book. We would also like to thank the publication team at McGraw Hill, particularly Rochelle Deighton and Martina Vascotto.

Shyamala would like to acknowledge the extreme patience shown by her husband and family for more than a year as she deserted them most weekends, writing and editing the cases and finding photos for case series. Shyamala would like to thank her longstanding Mohs technician, Jodie Wogoner, for her help with filing clinical images. Duncan would like to again acknowledge the forbearance of his family for this additional project. He knew Shyamala was the right person to lead this endeavour and he would like to thank her for her dedication, high standards and her friendship. Both of us would like to extend our sincere thanks to all of the patients who very kindly consented to their clinical photos being used in this book. Without this generosity of spirit, we could not transmit our knowledge to the next generation of doctors.

It is important also to acknowledge the debt we owe to our Dermatologic surgery mentors who have passed on their passion for teaching the next generation. In particular, Shyamala would like to thank Dudley Hill, Alastair Carruthers, Larry Warshawski and David Zloty. Duncan would like to thank Rob Paver, Shawn Richards, Howard Studniberg and Michelle Hunt.

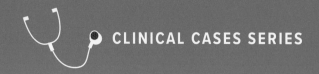

CLINICAL CASES SERIES

Clinical Cases in Dermatologic Surgery

SHYAMALA HUILGOL and DUNCAN STANFORD

Mc
Graw
Hill

NOTICE

Medicine is an ever-changing science. As new research and clinical experience broaden our knowledge, changes in treatment and drug therapy are required. The editors and the publisher of this work have checked with sources believed to be reliable in their efforts to provide information that is complete and generally in accord with the standards accepted at the time of publication. However, in view of the possibility of human error or changes in medical sciences, neither the editors, nor the publisher, nor any other party who has been involved in the preparation or publication of this work, warrant that the information contained herein is in every respect accurate or complete. Readers are encouraged to confirm the information contained herein with other sources. For example, and in particular, readers are advised to check the product information sheet included in the package of each drug they plan to administer to be certain that the information contained in this book is accurate and that changes have not been made in the recommended dose or in the contraindications for administration. This recommendation is of particular importance in connection with new or infrequently used drugs.

First edition published 2024

Copyright © 2024 McGraw Hill Education (Australia) Pty Ltd

Additional owners of copyright are acknowledged in on-page credits.

Every effort has been made to trace and acknowledge copyrighted material. The authors and publisher tender their apologies should any infringement have occurred.

Reproduction and communication for educational purposes

The Australian *Copyright Act 1968* (the Act) allows a maximum of one chapter or 10% of the pages of this work, whichever is the greater, to be reproduced and/or communicated by any educational institution for its educational purposes provided that the institution (or the body that administers it) has sent a Statutory Educational notice to Copyright Agency and been granted a licence. For details of statutory educational and other copyright licences contact: Copyright Agency, 66 Goulburn Street, Sydney NSW 2000. Telephone: (02) 9394 7600. Website: www.copyright.com.au

Reproduction and communication for other purposes

Apart from any fair dealing for the purposes of study, research, criticism or review, as permitted under the Act, no part of this publication may be reproduced, distributed or transmitted in any form or by any means, or stored in a database or retrieval system, without the written permission of McGraw Hill Education (Australia) Pty Ltd, including, but not limited to, any network or other electronic storage.

Enquiries should be made to the publisher via www.mheducation.com.au or marked for the attention of the permissions editor at the address below.

National Library of Australia Cataloguing-in-Publication Entry

A catalogue record for this work is available from the National Library of Australia

Authors: Shyamala Huilgol, Duncan Stanford
Title: Clinical cases in dermatologic surgery
Edition: 1st edition
ISBN: 9781760427313

Published in Australia by
McGraw Hill Education (Australia) Pty Ltd
Level 33, 680 George Street, Sydney NSW 2000
Publisher: Rochelle Deighton
Production manager: Martina Vascotto
Copyeditor: Julie Wicks
Proofreader: Meredith Lewin
Permissions manager: Rachel Norton
Cover design: Simon Rattray, Squirt Creative
Cover image: Shyamala Huilgol
Cover background image: fotograzia/Getty Images
Internal design: ChristaBella Designs
Typeset by Straive
Printed in Singapore by Markono Print Media Pte Ltd

Contents

CONTENTS

Preface

Clinical Cases in Dermatologic Surgery is envisaged as a very practical educational aid for all doctors practicing skin cancer surgery, particularly for the more difficult head and neck sites. The editors greatly enjoy teaching and have been instructing dermatology registrars and residents in similar advanced closure techniques for more than 25 years, along with teaching medical students and colleagues in other specialties. This book was first conceived by Duncan as a companion to the new second edition of *Dermatologic Surgery: A manual of defect repair options* (2023), which he edited together with contributing author, Leslie Storey, and in which Shyamala wrote a chapter on "Surgical complications and their management". We have followed the same order of site-based sections and chapters as in *Dermatologic Surgery* to assist with cross-referencing and we would highly recommend perusal of this comprehensive and practical textbook and its associated videos for greater detail in any area of interest. Although this book's origins are as a companion book, it is easily used as a standalone resource and may serve to "dip a toe" into advanced dermatologic surgery.

Clinical Cases in Dermatologic Surgery and *Dermatologic Surgery* are also published online on McGraw Hill's new AccessWorldMed website https://accessworldmed.mhmedical.com/.

The problem-based format that we chose for this book is based upon the *viva voce* final exams undertaken by dermatology registrars in Australia, but it is widely applicable in everyday clinical practice. In each case, readers are presented with a defect or tumour, and are asked three to five questions on management, including initial reconstruction, precautions, after-care, management of complications and revision. The cases in this book may be done in any order as they do not rely upon assumed knowledge from previous cases. However, readers may enjoy seeing different approaches to similar defects within each section. We recommend reading the question and formulating the answer before progressing to the answer. It is worth remembering that surgery is practiced by individuals and there may be more than one correct approach to the problem. We have attempted to discuss alternative approaches and give a balanced overview of the options. References have been kept to a minimum in this book, with a greater review of the literature found in *Dermatologic Surgery*.

Thank you for reading this book. We welcome feedback from readers.

Shyamala Huilgol and Duncan Stanford

About the authors

The Editors

Shyamala Claire Huilgol
MBBS(Hons), FACD, FACMS
Mohs Surgeon, Adelaide Skin and Eye Centre, South Australia, Australia
Clinical Professor, Department of Dermatology, Royal Adelaide Hospital and University of
Adelaide, South Australia, Australia

Duncan Stanford
MBBS, MSc(Med), FACD, FACMS
Mohs Surgeon, South Coast Dermatology, Kiama and Wollongong Day Surgery, Wollongong,
New South Wales, Australia
Clinical Associate Professor, University of Wollongong, New South Wales, Australia
Former Chief Examiner, Australasian College of Dermatologists

The Contributors

Paul Cherian MBBS(Hons), FACD, FACMS
Mohs surgeon, Dermatology Specialist Centre, Clayfield, QLD

Dougal Coates BSc, MBBS, FACD
Mohs surgeon, Princess Alexandra Hospital, QLD

Simon Harrington Lee MBBS, MMed, FACD, FACMS
Mohs surgeon, The Skin Hospital, Darlinghurst & Westmead, NSW

Karyn Lun MBBS, FACD, FACMS
Mohs surgeon, Queensland Institute of Dermatology, South Brisbane, QLD

Gilberto Moreno Bonilla MBBS(AMC), FACD
Mohs surgeon, The Skin Hospital, Westmead, NSW

Niamh Anna O'Sullivan MBBS, PhD, MRCS, FACD
Mohs surgeon, St Luke's Clinic, Potts Point, NSW

Tim Rutherford MBBS(Hons), FACD, FACMS
Mohs surgeon, Skin Health Institute, Carlton, VIC

Dinesh Selva MBBS (Hons), FRANZCO, DHSc
Oculoplastic surgeon, Royal Adelaide Hospital, Adelaide SA

Nicholas C Stewart BSc, MBBS, FACD
Mohs surgeon, The Skin Hospital, Darlinghurst & Westmead, NSW

Leslie Storey MD, FAAD, FACMS
Mohs surgeon, Valley Skin Institute, Fresno, California, United States of America

Jessica Tong MBBS, FRANZCO
Oculoplastic Fellow, Royal Adelaide Hospital, Adelaide, SA

Richard Turner MBBCh, FRCP
Mohs surgeon, Churchill Hospital, Oxford, United Kingdom

Edward Upjohn MBBS(Hons), MMed, FACD, FACMS
Mohs surgeon, Skin Health Institute, Carlton, VIC

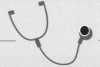

Section 1
The nose

Case 1
Ed Upjohn, Paul Cherian and Shyamala Huilgol

A 77-year-old man with a poorly defined nodular and infiltrating BCC of the central nose tip underwent Mohs surgery, giving a 13 × 15 mm defect (**Photo A**).

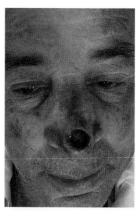

Photo A Post-Mohs surgery nose tip defect
Image courtesy of Shyamala Huilgol

QUESTION 1
What are your four favoured repair options?

Answer
1. Dorsal nasal rotation flap
2. Bilobed transposition flap
3. Myocutaneous flap: superiorly based
4. Full-thickness graft

Comment on alternatives
Primary closure will cause distortion. Second intention healing would likely leave a pale, shiny, depressed scar and risks distortion of the nostril rims. A split-thickness graft is a poor option.

QUESTION 2
Comment on the relative merits of nasal flaps versus full-thickness grafts.

Answer

Nasal flaps: Nasal tip skin is sebaceous, tightly bound to underlying muscle and visible in everyday life. Closure options include a local flap to recruit laxity from the upper nose or a full-thickness graft. In general, local flaps are preferred despite their complexity in design and execution, need for extensive undermining, postoperative swelling and bruising, and large scars because of more rapid healing and the ability to replace the defect with matching skin of the correct thickness. Nasal flaps are more robust than grafts, having the nasalis muscle in their pedicle, and may heal better than grafts in those with underlying illnesses.

Due to the sebaceous nature of nasal skin, scars may be noticeably indented, hence large flaps are best avoided in those with very sebaceous skin. Marked postoperative bruising and swelling may be poorly tolerated in the elderly and frail. When previous surgery or radiotherapy has compromised the blood supply, a flap may be risky.

Nasal flaps may lift the nasal tip, often cosmetically positive in the elderly, as long as the nares are not unnaturally visible on frontal view. The nose tip may also be flattened by flaps, particularly when the distal closure is across the nose tip. Twisting of the nose or pulling upon the nostril rims may result in other distortions, usually due to poor design or execution. Internal nasal valve compromise is a relatively common complication of flap surgery.

Full-thickness grafts: This is an excellent option in the elderly and frail, those taking anticoagulants, or when previous surgery or radiotherapy prevents further flap surgery. It is a relatively simple and one-stage procedure.

Graft colour and texture match may be difficult — the donor site should be chosen to match the colour and sebaceous nature of tip skin, which varies greatly. In less sebaceous noses, pre- or postauricular skin may be a good match, although fine hair may be troublesome. Preauricular skin is more sebaceous but often yellowish, while postauricular skin is usually thinner, with pink or brown tones. More sebaceous skin is also found on the nasolabial folds, forehead and submental area but may leave obvious scars in the first two of these donor sites. The conchal bowl has a good colour and texture match but the donor site is slow to heal by second intention with occasional prolonged tenderness. Grafts tend to develop hyperpigmentation with UV exposure – prevention requires strict sun protection for 3 months following healing.

Grafts may have a noticeable step or indentation at their margins. Measures to reduce this include:

- undermining the recipient site margins
- correct graft sizing
- thinning the graft to sit just below the surrounding skin (making the defect deeper isn't a good option on the nose tip as cartilage will be exposed)
- "ship-to-shore" differential suturing aids exact placement of the graft relative to the surrounding tissue
- fenestration and pexing of the graft to drain haemoserous fluid and prevent central festooning
- a firm external bolus/bolster postoperatively to prevent fluid build-up
- post-healing application of firm pressure for 5–10 minutes at a time through the day to reduce oedema and swelling.

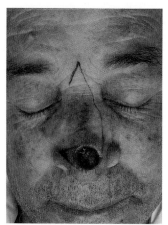

Photo B Dorsal nasal rotation flap with back-cut design. Note favourable placement of closure lines in cosmetic junction lines— alar crease and dorsum/sidewall junction.
Image courtesy of Shyamala Huilgol

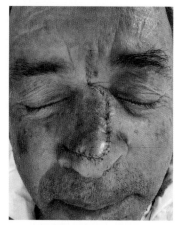

Photo C Flap closure
Image courtesy of Shyamala Huilgol

Minor failure is common, particularly near nostril rims, and may lead to graft contraction and distortion of the nostrils. Complete graft necrosis due to haematoma or infection may occur. Grafts require a vascularised bed and may not be placed on bare cartilage. This problem may be overcome by placing a muscle flap in the base of the wound, then grafting over it.

QUESTION 3

The dorsal nasal rotation flap in **Photo B** is performed. What are the potential pitfalls of this repair?

Answer

The flap extends through the natural concavity of the nasal root and may lead to its blunting and tenting of the scar across this area.

The recruited skin above the defect is often thicker than that below the defect, hence there may be a noticeable step at the distal nose tip scar, along with an impression of flap bulkiness. These may need later laser resurfacing or surgical revision. The scar across the nose tip may indent, a common problem in sebaceous skin. In this case, it has been possible to favourably place the majority of other nasal scar lines in cosmetic junction lines (**Photo C**), largely avoiding the centre line.

The flap may flatten nasal tip projection or lead to nasal tip and alar asymmetry through torsion. Hence, flap design and execution are crucial in permitting free rotation of the dorsal nasal skin and muscle, and the closure of the correcting Burow's triangle. In our case, there is some mild postoperative distortion, with the right nostril rim pushed downwards and the left pulled upwards: both resolved with time (**Photos D and E**). This flap has also very slightly lifted the nose tip, a favourable effect. Internal nasal valve function may be compromised in patients with poorly supported alar arches.

Indentation of nasal scars is common with flaps, particularly on the sebaceous tip area. Preventive measures include placement in cosmetic junction lines, undermining of primary and secondary defects, pexing sutures to prevent trapdooring, precise matching of levels on either side and eversion of suture lines with buried sutures. Postoperative measures include compression, treatment of trapdooring with IL steroids, subcision and laser resurfacing. On occasion, surgical debulking may be required.

The extensive undermining of the nose results in substantial postoperative bruising and may make future flap surgery more difficult.

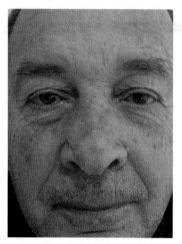 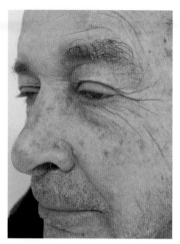

Photos D and E Excellent result at 3 months with frontal and left side views. Patient will compress mild bulkiness of the right side; he declined IL triamcinolone.
Image courtesy of Shyamala Huilgol

QUESTION 4

What could be done if the scar from the back-cut incision was noticeably thickened or causing webbing?

Answer

Compression and time may fix the issue. Intralesional triamcinolone acetonide (0.3–0.8 mL of 10 mg/mL) may be given at the 6-week postoperative mark and repeated monthly as needed. If unsuccessful, Z-plasty revision (**Photos F and G**) may give excellent improvement.

Extension of the rotation arc or extending the back-cut are preventive options during the design stage. Scars on the nasal bridge can be "stress tested" at the time of closure by raising the eyebrows and opening the mouth. (Sitting the patient up is also helpful, but usually impractical.) This will place the scar under maximum tension, allowing early identification and immediate treatment of this issue with a Z-plasty or plasties.

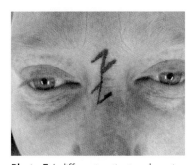

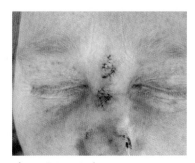

Photo F A different patient undergoing 45° Z-plasty revision for persistent sensation of tightness when raising eyebrows, occurring in bilobed flap scar across the nasal root
Image courtesy of Shyamala Huilgol

Photo G Post Z-plasty revision. Resolution of problem was achieved at subsequent 3-month review.
Image courtesy of Shyamala Huilgol

Case 2
Paul Cherian and Shyamala Huilgol

Consider the two nose tip defects following Mohs surgery clearance of BCCs in **Photos A and B.**

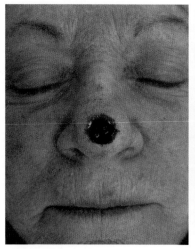

Photo A Central nasal tip defect measuring 10 × 12 mm
Image courtesy of Shyamala Huilgol

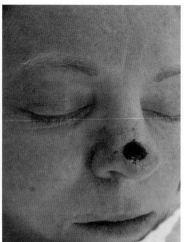

Photo B Right nose tip defect measuring 8 × 10 mm
Image courtesy of Shyamala Huilgol

QUESTION 1
List four reconstructive options for these nasal tip defects.

Answer
1. Myocutaneous flap
2. Bilobed flap
3. Dorsal nasal rotation (Rieger) flap
4. Full-thickness skin graft

QUESTION 2

Discuss the advantages and disadvantages for myocutaneous and bilobed flaps, including the prevention and treatment of problems.

Answer

Both flaps have the advantage of recruitment of similar-appearing skin, the ability to match the defect depth through excision of residual nasalis muscle in the defect, and robust vascularity due to inclusion of nasalis muscle.

They commonly suffer from post-surgical telangiectasia, which is exacerbated by preexisting rosacea and may be treated with vascular laser or IPL.

1. Myocutaneous flap: superiorly or laterally based

Advantages:

- Good reach to the tip and nostril rims when correctly mobilised, especially the superiorly based flap.
- Laterally based flap preserves the alar groove, hides incision line in this cosmetic junction line and avoids crossing the midline.

Disadvantages:

- Execution is challenging for the inexperienced.
- Risks of step-off or contour mismatch — reduced by excising nasalis from defect base; undermining the defect; and using everting dermal sutures at the flap's advancing edge.
- Pincushioning — minimised by these same measures plus regular compression to the flap, commencing 2 weeks post surgery.
- Distal flap necrosis — ensure minimal flap tension, usually requires horizontal incisional release of nasalis in superiorly based flap; avoid damage to nasalis and blood vessels during undermining; avoid this flap in individuals where the nasalis is underdeveloped. The blood supply through the muscle-only nasalis pedicle is less reliable than combined cutaneous and muscular pedicles and the flap does occasionally fail.
- Downward displacement or "bullnosing" of the ala and nostril rim with rotation/advancement of the flap — requires careful design and execution; may need later revision.

- Internal nasal valve compromise — must be discussed preoperatively as it is relatively common; helped by postoperative IL steroids and compression.
- Haematoma — careful haemostasis (more difficult in the double-pedicle variant); BIPP intranasal packing for 24–48 hours, especially for those on anticoagulants.

2 Bilobed transposition flap — laterally based

Advantages:
- Fullness of primary lobe is often helpful in re-creating the natural nose tip contour.
- The curvilinear scars "confuse the eye" and are less noticeable than one might expect.
- Unlikely to cause secondary movement of free margins when correctly designed and executed.

Disadvantages:
- Design and execution are difficult for the inexperienced.
- Pincushioning of primary lobe — minimised by correct lobe sizing; matching depth of the primary lobe to defect; a pexing suture from the undersurface of flap to the defect's base; everting sutures and compression as discussed earlier. This problem potentially requires multiple steroid injections or further surgery to debulk the flap. Laser resurfacing or dermabrasion is a helpful final revision.
- Distal flap necrosis — include the nasalis in the flap and avoid trimming it to match the defect's depth.
- Nasal valve compromise — a suspension suture may be used intra-operatively; IL steroids postoperatively; or surgical revision.
- Torsion of nasal tip or ala — precise design and execution, including closure of the correcting Burow's triangle is essential. Ensure that the tension vector for closure of the triangle is perpendicular to the free margin.
- Multiple cosmetic units required for recruitment (nasal tip, dorsum and sidewall) and scars may cross the midline.

QUESTION 3

Describe how you would perform a superiorly based myocutaneous flap with a single muscular pedicle.

Answer

1. Design the triangular flap with a vertical long axis, ensuring that the width of the defect and the flap adjacent to the defect are equal.
2. Excise residual nasalis muscle from the defect's base.
3. Carefully incise the more lateral margin of the flap, staying *above* the nasalis musculature, then undermine *above* the nasalis to the nasofacial sulcus. Obtain haemostasis.
4. Deeply incise the medial aspect of the flap through nasalis muscle, then undermine the flap *beneath* the nasalis to the nasofacial sulcus. Obtain haemostasis.
5. Assess flap movement with a skin hook — in most cases one needs to incise the nasalis horizontally at the superior aspect.
6. Undermine both the leading edge of the flap to allow movement into the defect and the margins of the defect to allow eversion of the defect edges.
7. Close the defect with 5-0 Monosyn® (or similar) at the advancing edge of the flap (key suture). Ensure eversion without excessive tension, which may compromise flap vascularity. The geometry of the advancing edge of the flap may need to be trimmed to exactly fit the recipient defect. Sometimes, it is better to slightly enlarge the defect to match the flap.

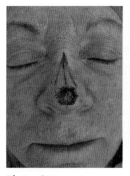 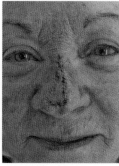 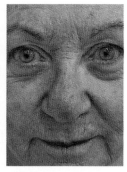

Photo C Myocutaneous flap design
Image courtesy of Shyamala Huilgol

Photo D Myocutaneous flap closure
Image courtesy of Shyamala Huilgol

Photo E Outcome at 10 months, following erbium laser resurfacing and one full-face IPL with further IPL planned
Image courtesy of Shyamala Huilgol

8. Secure the flap with further buried sutures. Pay attention to the vectors of tension to avoid nasal tip torsion or alar elevation.

9. Approximate the epidermis with 6-0 Dafilon® (or similar).

QUESTION 4

Describe how you would perform a Zitelli-variant bilobed transposition flap.

Answer

For a medial nose tip defect, the flap is generally laterally based.

1. Draw a Burow's or apex triangle from the lateral lower edge of the defect, with a 30-degree apical angle and, if possible, placed in the alar crease. Measure from the apex to the furthest point of the defect and draw an arc of that radius ("diameter arc"). Draw a parallel but smaller arc from the mid-point of the defect ("radius arc").

2. Construct a line extending 45° from the apex triangle. The primary lobe of the flap is drawn from the junction of the defect and lower radial arc, the tip of the lobe then meets the diameter arc line and curves back to the radius arc. The width of this lobe equals the width of the primary defect, and is bisected by the 45° line.

3. Draw a line at 90° to the apex triangle. Construct the secondary lobe, beginning at the termination point of the primary lobe arc, extending to the diameter arc and back down to the radius arc. This lobe is about two-thirds the primary defect's width. Triangulate the secondary lobe's point to form a Burow's triangle with a 30° angle, lying on the 90° line.

4. Excise the *apical* Burow's triangle down to the subnasalis plane and reserve in case of need. Incise the primary and secondary lobes (including the triangulation) beneath the nasalis.

5. Undermine the flap and edges of the primary defect in the subnasalis plane, paying particular attention to the point of pivotal restraint around the apex triangle. Check flap mobility. Achieve meticulous haemostasis.

6. Transpose the primary lobe into the primary defect, and the secondary lobe into the secondary defect. Suture the tertiary defect closed first, then the primary lobe in position, using 5-0 Monosyn™ or similar.

7. Check the internal nasal valve patency by physically occluding the contralateral nostril and asking the patient to breathe in and out. If correction is needed, sutures closing the primary lobe will need to be removed. The suspensory suture is placed in the supramucosal tissue of the defect. The desired vector of tension is determined by again blocking the contralateral nares, pulling superior-laterally on the inserted suture (opening the internal nasal valve), then asking which position (lateral or superior-lateral) allows maximal nasal inflow. Once the best vector has been determined, the suture is passed back into the flap (a visible dermal dimple is seen) and tied off. Usually, this will be just superior to the apex of the Burow's triangle. If the flap blanches post suture insertion, the suture must be removed and reinserted. In very floppy or large defects, the suture is laterally anchored to medial maxillary periosteum/deep tissues.

8. Suture the secondary lobe into position, and trim any excess tissue resulting from the Burow's triangle. Place 6-0 cutaneous Dafilon™ sutures.

9. Insert intranasal BIPP gauze for 24–48 hours to minimise sub-flap haematoma formation.

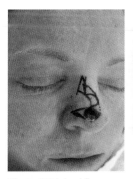

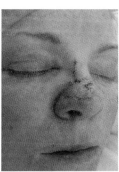

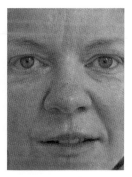

Photo F Bilobed flap design with Zitelli modification
Image courtesy of Shyamala Huilgol

Photo G Bilobed flap closure
Image courtesy of Shyamala Huilgol

Photo H Outcome at one year, following erbium laser resurfacing and IPL
Image courtesy of Shyamala Huilgol

Case 3
Leslie Storey and Shyamala Huilgol

An 82-year-old man with an ulcerated nose tip BCC required four stages of Mohs surgery, giving a 33 × 27 mm defect with cartilage at the base (**Photo A**).

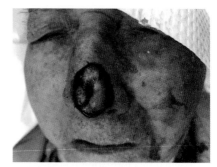

Photo A Nose tip defect
Image courtesy of Leslie Storey

QUESTION 1
What are the closure options for this defect? Discuss their advantages and disadvantages.

Answer

A full-thickness skin graft is commonly used for nasal tip defects. Its chief advantage is avoiding tissue rearrangement. Hence, it is helpful when the defect is too large for local flap closure, when previous surgery makes a local flap problematic, and in the elderly and frail where a large flap may be poorly tolerated. There may be difficulties in obtaining a good colour, texture and contour match and there is greater potential for failure than a flap. Partial or complete failure is more likely in larger grafts, near the nostril rim, when there is underlying cartilage, in smokers and in the presence of underlying systemic disease.

The well-vascularised paramedian forehead flap is a reliable method for repairing large nose defects, particularly on the nose tip and for more complex full-thickness defects. It usually provides a good contour and colour match, with a less sebaceous texture than the nose tip. However, there is a 2 to 3-week period with a pedicle which requires dressing care and limits normal activities (glasses cannot be worn) and then a second, flap division procedure. Many patients benefit from further revision to thin and refine the nose tip contour and to the forehead donor scar, which varies in quality. The flap is very dependent on the patient's forehead and scalp skin being of good quality, with sufficient laxity, and preferably not hair-bearing (later laser hair removal is possible). Prior radiotherapy or significant surgery to the forehead will compromise the vascular supply and are contraindications.

Comment on alternatives
The defect was too large for local or two-stage nasolabial flaps.

QUESTION 2
You elect to do a paramedian forehead flap, given the larger defect size, underlying cartilage and proximity to the nostril rim. Describe steps in flap design, naming the artery and any measures you would consider with a history of heavy smoking and/or diabetes.

Answer
1. Make an exact template of the defect (e.g. with suture packet). Consider enlarging the defect to encompass the entire cosmetic subunit (e.g. nose tip) to hide junction lines.
2. Assess the forehead donor skin. The contralateral side is preferred for easier flap rotation, but the ipsilateral side may be used if the tissue match is superior.
3. Palpate and then mark the contralateral supratrochlear artery and a 12–15 mm pedicle base width around it. If a history of heavy smoking or diabetes exists, consider using Doppler ultrasound to confirm patency of the artery to the midforehead. If there are concerns, assess the ipsilateral artery as this may also be used.
4. Measure the distance from the pedicle base to the distal defect, using a non-stretch material, rotate onto the forehead and mark out an arc, allowing some extra length (approximately 10 mm) for rotational shortening. Place the template on the forehead with the distal border aligned with the arc, draw around it and connect this circular shape to

the marked pedicle base. Consider angling the distal flap towards the midline to obtain extra length and avoid hair-bearing skin.

5. Double-check your measurements and flap design.

QUESTION 3
Describe specific complications and their management.

Answer

Vascular compromise

If the flap is pale, cool and fails to blanch with pressure, arterial compromise must be remedied. A dark purple colour indicates venous compromise. Look for vascular compromise, starting proximally and reassessing each measure after several minutes before proceeding.

1. Remove all dressings.
2. Reposition flap base to remove any kinking.
3. Remove sutures closing the secondary defect at the pedicle base.
4. Remove sutures from the distal flap. It may be resutured at a later date.

Persistent arterial compromise will require complete flap take down, followed as necessary by replacement in its original site. Failure to recover indicates arterial damage and is likely not salvageable. However, it should be reviewed over one week to see if it can be saved. If the flap fails, one based on the remaining supratrochlear artery may be used.

For venous compromise that persists after the initial measures, conservative management is reasonable: hourly ice packs for 48 hours (when awake) and then review.

Pincushioning or trapdooring

Undermining the defect at the time of flap division, excising excessive granulation tissue from the defect base, thinning the flap and freshening both defect and flap edges assist in prevention. Later, IL triamcinolone acetonide, subcision and laser resurfacing, in that order, may be helpful. Surgical revision is sometimes needed.

Bulkiness

Thinning of the flap at the time of division is tricky as over-thinning can lead to necrosis, while not enough predictably leads to a bulky flap. The measures described earlier to counter trapdooring are helpful in shaping the upper portion of the flap but the distal flap may well require surgical revision. Always inform patients that a third procedure may be needed. Consider IL triamcinolone before revisional surgery.

Obvious scar lines

Replacing the entire cosmetic subunit helps in prevention. Later, dermabrasion or laser resurfacing are useful.

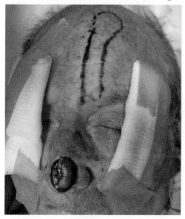

Photo B Forehead flap design
Image courtesy of Leslie Storey

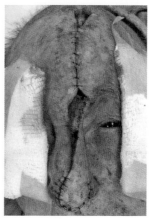

Photo C Forehead flap sutured in place
Image courtesy of Leslie Storey

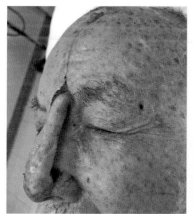

Photo D Forehead flap prior to division at 3 weeks
Image courtesy of Leslie Storey

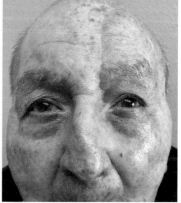

Photo E Long-term outcome at 3 months with excellent restoration of nose tip contour and colour. Depressed vertical flap donor scar on forehead is usual as it is under tension. The superior area that underwent healing by second intention has also done well
Image courtesy of Leslie Storey

Case 4
Duncan Stanford

A 60-year-old female has an 8 × 9 mm defect on the left ala (**Photo A**) after infiltrating BCC was cleared in one stage by Mohs micrographic surgery.

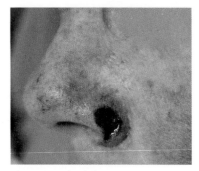

Photo A Mohs defect
Image courtesy of Duncan Stanford

QUESTION 1
List your three preferred repair options.

Answer
1. Second intention healing
2. Bilobed transposition flap (medial base)
3. Full-thickness skin graft (conchal or other sebaceous skin donor site)
4. Spiral alar flap

Comment
Any of these four would be good choices. See below for discussion of second intention healing.

A medially based bilobed flap is an effective and popular single-stage option if well designed and executed. Pincushioning of the lower lobe is common but responds well to intralesional steroid.

A full-thickness skin graft from the conchal bowl (left to heal by second intent) is a good choice but there will be prolonged donor site wound care. Glabellar crease and nasolabial fold donor sites also provide an excellent tissue match, but the facial scars and reduced fullness of the cheek may sometimes be obvious. The preauricular skin is often too yellow but sometimes provides an excellent colour and texture match.

A spiral rotation flap needs careful design for this defect on the alar rim, away from the alar crease and with a horizontal orientation. An intra-alar design would risk alar lift; extending to the nasal sidewall would be best, but then it will not be possible to conceal the scar in the alar crease.

Comment on alternatives

A nasolabial transposition flap will require enlargement of the defect to reach the alar groove and will blunt the alar crease to at least some extent. Primary repair is a poor option. Composite grafts with skin and cartilage are best reserved for deeper, full-thickness defects, along the nostril rim. A nasolabial interpolation (two-stage) flap is a larger procedure, and unlikely to look better than a full-thickness skin graft.

QUESTION 2

The patient elects to allow healing by second intention. What are the advantages and disadvantages of that approach?

Answer

Advantages

- Shallow defect suitable as contraction with alar rim notching is less likely to occur
- Simple option requiring no further surgery or sutures to remove
- Avoids extra risks and complications of more complex repairs
- Scarring confined to the area but smaller than defect due to contraction of about 30%
- The alar groove and crease are always prone to blunting from flap repairs with loss of normal well-defined cosmetic unit junction lines
- Flap repairs commonly result in some degree of internal nasal valve constriction
- Colour of the scar is likely to be as good as a full-thickness graft in this fair-skinned patient

Disadvantages
- Defect closer to alar rim than ideal and risks free margin contraction, with alar rim notching
- Daily wound care of an open wound required for around 4 weeks
- Hypopigmented and indented scar may result
- Infection is more common than after a sutured repair but still unlikely

Comment

In defects that are deeper, a "guiding" suture can be placed or a piece of cartilage inserted into the open base to prevent alar rim distortion as second intention healing progresses.

QUESTION 3

What instructions would you give the patient about wound care?

Answer

The preferred approach will vary somewhat between experienced practitioners.

A non-stick pressure dressing is applied over white soft petrolatum and is left intact and dry for 24–48 hours. (Some dermatologic surgeons still prefer antibiotic ointment, in which case contact allergy risk must be discussed.) Tell the patient to avoid bending over and heavy lifting for 48 hours and to apply hourly ice packs for 10–15 mins on day 1 to reduce swelling and bleeding risk. Discomfort should be minimal. Provide a written wound care sheet describing signs of infection, how to manage bleeding with ice packs and contact details in case of concerns.

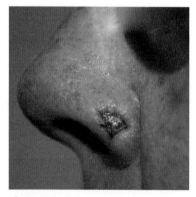

Photo B Healing at 1 week showing appropriate granulation and minimal contraction

Image courtesy of Duncan Stanford

The wound should be cleaned daily with saline (e.g. a teaspoon of salt in a cup of cooled boiled water) or 3% hydrogen peroxide. Petrolatum should be reapplied with a non-stick dressing. A wound check at 1 week is ideal for reassurance (**Photo B**). After this, it is easier to use a hydrocolloid dressing (e.g. Duoderm Thin®) every few days as this accelerates healing and looks better. This should be stopped if overgranulation occurs. Review again at 6 weeks to assess any potential cosmetic issues or deal with delayed healing.

QUESTION 4

What complication is evident at 10 weeks (see **Photos C** and **D**) and how might it be treated if the patient was concerned?

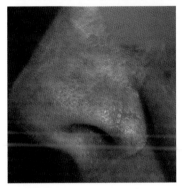

Photo C Side view at 10 weeks
Image courtesy of Duncan Stanford

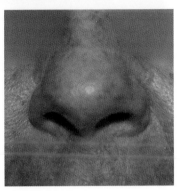

Photo D Front view at 10 weeks
Image courtesy of Duncan Stanford

Answer

The patient has an indented scar.

These respond well to resurfacing procedures—laser resurfacing with an Er:YAG or CO_2 laser or manual dermabrasion.

Comment

The depression due to the scar is less impactful here than asymmetry of a flap with alar groove blunting or colour and contour issues from a full-thickness graft. This patient was very pleased with the cosmetic outcome and she found the wound care straightforward and tolerable.

Case 5
Leslie Storey and Shyamala Huilgol

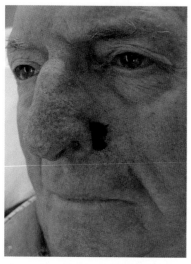

A 76-year-old man underwent Mohs surgery for a nodular BCC in the alar groove with a final complex alar, medial cheek and cutaneous upper lip defect measuring 10 × 15 mm (**Photo A**).

Photo A Post-Mohs surgery defect
Image courtesy of Shyamala Huilgol

QUESTION 1
List three closure options in order of preference.

Answer

1. Shark island pedicle flap
2. Advancement flap along nasolabial fold and full-thickness graft to ala
3. Second intention healing

QUESTION 2
What are the pros and cons for each closure?

Answer
1. **Shark island pedicle flap.** This is the repair of choice as it restores all three units and their junction lines with matching and robust tissue in a one-stage procedure. The trapdooring of the alar portion of the flap is usually desirable in re-creating the natural fullness of the ala, but may require intralesional steroid injections. The flap is more complex to design and execute.
2. **Advancement flap along nasolabial fold with full-thickness graft to ala.** This repair divides the defect into two sections with separate repairs in order to maintain the demarcation between the nose and adjacent cheek and lip. The advancement flap scar will be hidden within the natural lines of the nasolabial fold with the dog ear curving around the alar groove to the nasal sill. Care must be taken to anchor the flap with a pexing suture to prevent lateral pull upon the ala. The graft has the usual risks of failure to take and a poor match. (The Burow's triangle will likely have hair so is not a good option for the graft.)
3. **Second intention.** This has the major advantage of simplicity but at the cost of longer healing. The scar will be well-placed in the alar groove but may be quite white and there is the possibility of alar and upper lip distortion through scar contraction.

Comment on repair
This is a difficult defect to reconstruct as it spans three central facial cosmetic units with very well-defined junctions; hence, any distortions will be quite obvious.

Comment on alternatives
Primary closure is not possible without distortion of the ala and nasolabial fold. A full-thickness graft will be very unattractive as it will cross the cosmetic units. A nasolabial transposition flap is also a poor option, blunting the lateral portion of the alar groove.

QUESTION 3

Describe the design and execution of the shark island flap.

Answer

The shark island flap is a "Pac-man" variant of the island pedicle flap, with a larger upper jaw or "snout" and smaller lower jaw swinging together to close the "mouth" and re-create the alar groove[1]. It has an interesting 3D construction in which the snout portion sits at a right angle to the plane of the main portion of the flap.

1. Measure the horizontal width of the alar portion of the defect and mark the high point of the flap's "snout" this same distance above the defect. Measure the vertical height of the alar portion of the defect and draw the same length laterally from the previously marked high point of the "snout". Draw the triangular island pedicle flap from the lateral aspect of the "snout" and the inferior border of the cutaneous lip defect. Mark the nasolabial fold; it will be advanced upwards within the flap to return to its usual high point at the upper alar groove (see **Photo B**).

2. Use an infra-orbital block, then local anaesthesia infiltration. Using sterile technique, incise the flap, freeing the snout at its depth but taking care to maintain the snout's myocutaneous pedicle by preserving deep muscular tissue on its underside. Free the tail of the flap completely at its depth in the nasolabial fold to increase mobility and undermine the leading edge of the cheek portion of the island pedicle flap by approximately 5 mm. Undermine the defect, the skin surrounding the flap and possibly a small amount at the flap margins. Obtain haemostasis.

3. Place the key buried suture from the "snout" of the flap into the inferior border of the alar defect, then continue suturing the snout into the medial border of the alar defect. The flap should move into place, with the jaws of the shark closing and re-creating the alar groove. Consider placing a buried suture from the undersurface of the leading edge of the flap to the depth of the alar groove to prevent trapdooring, but be cautious with this and avoid compromising the flap's viability. Use fine cutaneous sutures only (no deep sutures) to close the "mouth" of the shark, forming the new alar groove. Continue placing buried sutures to suture the remainder of the flap into place and close the secondary defect behind the flap. Place cutaneous sutures (**Photo C**) and arrange review at 3 months (**Photos D and E**).

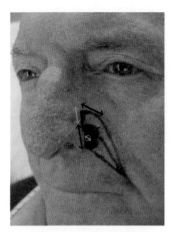

Photo B Design of flap. Width of alar portion of the defect is equal to the height of the snout (light blue), while height of the alar portion of the defect is equal to the length of the snout (purple). Key suture is from midpoint of the blue line to midpoint of the inferior alar portion of the defect.
Image courtesy of Shyamala Huilgol

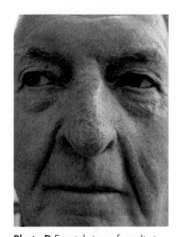

Photo D Frontal view of result at 3 months. Excellent restoration of contour and symmetry. Note that the groove above and parallel to the nasolabial fold was pre-existing and is apparent in Photo A.
Image courtesy of Shyamala Huilgol

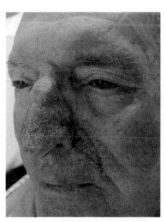

Photo C Flap sutured in place
Image courtesy of Shyamala Huilgol

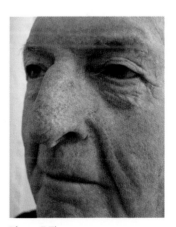

Photo E Three-quarter view at 3 months
Image courtesy of Shyamala Huilgol

Reference

1. Cvancara JL, Wentzell JM. Shark island pedicle flap for repair of combined nasal ala-perialar defects. Dermatol Surg 2006; 32(5): 726–729.

Case 6
Dougal Coates

A 55-year-old woman presented with an infiltrative BCC on the midline of her dorsal nose. The tumour was cleared in two Mohs surgery stages with a final defect of 14 × 18 mm (**Photo A**).

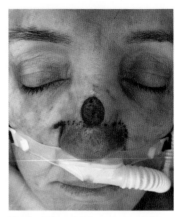

Photo A Post-Mohs surgery defect
Image courtesy of Dougal Coates

QUESTION 1
What are your three favoured repair options? Comment on their relative merits.

Answer
1. Bilateral advancement flap (O–T, A–T)
2. Paired V–Y subcutaneous island pedicle flaps
3. Full-thickness skin graft

Comment
The available laxity is lateral (nasal sidewall/medial cheek) and superior (nasal root/glabella) to this defect. Flap repairs using the lateral reservoir

may be incised along the alar crease, concealing the surgical scar at the junction of the nasal sidewall and alar cosmetic subunits. Utilising nasal root/glabella for defects of the lower dorsal nose requires an incisional reach, which is not always easily concealed.

1. A bilateral advancement flap (**Photo B**) is effective at repairing medium-sized defects of the dorsal nose, especially when the defect is at, or close to, the midline. Incisions are favourably hidden in the alar creases and also in the midline, another reliably good placement site for nasal scars. The flap is myocutaneous with submuscular undermining, providing a robust vascular supply with protection against flap necrosis and failure. In recruiting medial cheek laxity, tenting across the nasofacial sulcus is prevented with an absorbable pexing suture from the middle of the underside of the flap into the nasofacial sulcus (**Photo C**). Closure of the secondary defect along the alar crease may result in both tip and alar elevation, but this is usually temporary.

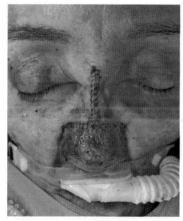

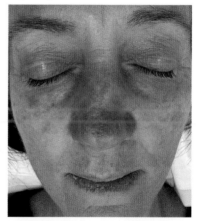

Photo B Repair closure with O – T flap. Note Burow's triangles in alar grooves.
Image courtesy of Dougal Coates

Photo C Excellent postoperative result at 3 months
Image courtesy of Dougal Coates

2. The tails of the paired V–Y subcutaneous island pedicle flaps are released from the medial cheek. Therefore, the flaps move into the defect without pulling on this site of origin, avoiding tenting across the nasofacial sulcus and also the secondary nose tip and alar elevation seen in the O–T repair. However, the superior incision lines do not fall into cosmetic junction lines, creating the potential for both visible triangular scars and pincushioning.

3. A full-thickness skin graft will fill the defect without tension, thus avoid distorting nasal structures, including the free margins of the nostrils. The obvious and most common complication is a mismatch in colour and/or contour. Many reasonable donor sites exist, including preauricular, postauricular, glabella (particularly for sebaceous nasal skin), nasofacial sulcus, upper forehead, neck, supraclavicular and arm. The most appropriate match must be tailored to the patient, with consideration given to the colour, degree of photodamage, thickness, texture and presence of terminal hairs, as well as ability to repair the donor site without morbidity.

For nasal defects with bone or cartilage denuded of periosteum or perichondrium (**Photo D**), a muscular flap may be used in conjunction with a full-thickness graft to provide both a well-vascularised bed and volume restoration. When options for a single-stage local flap are limited, such muscular flaps provide an alternative to multi-staged reconstructions. In this repair (**Photo E**), a Burow's triangle was excised superiorly to partially close the defect, as well as expose and recruit nasalis muscle, which was then advanced into the defect. The excised skin was utilised as a well-matched graft (**Photo F**). Nasalis muscle may also be used in a hinge flap: freed on three sides and at the depth, then folding over the remaining side into the defect, like the page of a book.

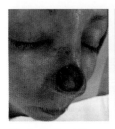 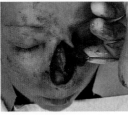 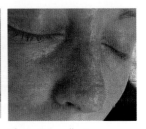

Photo D Nasal tip defect with exposed cartilage
Image courtesy of Dougal Coates

Photo E Superior Burow's triangle excised and saved for subsequent grafting. Left nasalis muscle mobilised and elevated with skin hook, prior to advancement into the nose tip defect.
Image courtesy of Dougal Coates

Photo F Excellent postoperative result at 3 months
Image courtesy of Dougal Coates

Comment on alternatives

There is not as much donor skin between the defect and glabella as is usually preferred for a dorsal nasal rotation back-cut flap. This repair will also require incision across the concavity of the nasal root, potentially causing some tenting or blunting. The defect is too high on the nose for a myocutaneous flap based on the nasalis or a bilobed flap repair.

QUESTION 2

A bilateral advancement flap is performed. At removal of sutures on day 6, you notice that the flap has undergone tip necrosis. What is your immediate management?

Answer

It's important to appreciate that the flap and tissue loss may be only superficial. Hence, supportive measures should be put in place, with the expectation that much of the flap will still be viable. Aggressive debridement at this point may both remove a natural and effective biologic dressing and also traumatise viable tissue, deepening the injury. Sutures are best left in place to avoid dislodging fragile tissue or permitting dehiscence. Swabs should be taken to exclude an occult or contributory infection, but empiric oral antibiotics are not typically necessary. Simple measures such as daily normal saline cleansing followed by liberal application of white soft petrolatum and a non-stick dressing over the necrotic area may be instituted, with close follow-up (twice weekly) and careful debridement of any superficial slough as needed. Enzymatic debridement (e.g. Flaminal® Hydro) may be helpful to conservatively manage a sloughy wound.

QUESTION 3

At 8 weeks following the procedure, the necrosed flap tip has healed into an irregular, atrophic central scar with erythema and telangiectasia. The patient is unhappy with the outcome. Discuss your options.

Answer

Firstly, the patient should be reassured that in the context of wound healing, 8 weeks post procedure is still very early in the overall remodelling of the wound. Explain that even with no active treatment, the cosmetic result will continue to improve over 6–12 months.

The usual practice is to wait until at least 3 months following complete healing before undertaking surgical revision. Silicone gel and sunblock should be used during this phase of conservative management and it is also helpful to review the patient regularly to provide support. Photos of similar issues and the eventual outcome provide useful information and reassurance. At 3 months, revisional techniques may include one or more of the following:

1. Further surgery
   a. Incising along the alar creases bilaterally, mobilising the previous flap and re-suturing.
   b. Performing conservative but complete and shallow excision of the atrophic scar, and repairing the defect with a full-thickness skin graft.

2. Laser
   a. Ablative laser (CO_2, erbium:YAG): very lightly to the atrophic scar and more deeply to the immediate surrounding skin, fading away from this point into the remainder of the cosmetic unit to reduce the visible step and feather any contrast with the surrounding skin. It should always be explained that there will be some degree of long-term hypopigmentation in the lasered area but that its visibility is reduced by the feathering and treatment of the entire cosmetic unit. Sun protection and avoidance must be meticulous for 3 months post ablation to prevent hyperpigmentation.
   b. Vascular laser (Nd:YAG, PDL, KTP) or IPL to treat the scar erythema and telangiectasia.

3. Needle subcision (e.g. 18 gauge BD Nokor™ admix): this often requires 2–3 treatments at monthly intervals to cut through any tethering from the undersurface of the scar to deeper tissue.

4. Injection of filler under scar: this would require re-injection every 6–12 months to maintain the improvement in contour.

A 56-year-old man underwent Mohs surgery of a biopsy-proven infiltrating BCC on the left nasal sidewall, resulting in a defect of 10 × 12 mm (**Photos A and B**).

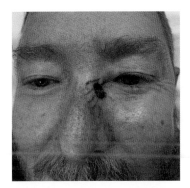

Photo A Post-Mohs surgery defect
Image courtesy of Paul Cherian

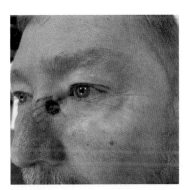

Photo B Post-Mohs surgery defect
Image courtesy of Paul Cherian

QUESTION 1

What are your three favoured repair options? Comment on their relative merits.

Answer

1. Rhombic transposition flap. A robust flap with matching skin from the adjacent glabellar cosmetic unit and placement of the secondary defect scar in preexisting rhytid line. See **Photos C and D**.

2. An inferiorly based O–L advancement flap with the dog ear in the medial canthus. This robust flap would use very similar skin and

place the scars in cosmetic junction lines and natural rhytids. It would require careful pexing to the nose to prevent downwards pull and eyelid distortion.

3. A full-thickness skin graft. This would work well here due to the relatively superficial nature of the defect, the nasalis muscle base and the ability to avoid encroaching further on medial canthal structures. The major issues are ensuring good take and obtaining a good colour and contour match.

Comment on alternatives

Other options include:

- A medially based bilobed transposition flap with secondary and tertiary lobes in the nasal root and glabella will produce a non-geometric scar in the midline that doesn't sit in existing rhytids.

- A transposed island pedicle flap from the glabella has a higher probability of pincushioning and is best for deeper defects.

- A glabella-based back-cut rotation flap has the key disadvantage of the scar line crossing the midline of the nose with potential for webbing and interference with the bridge of the patient's spectacles.

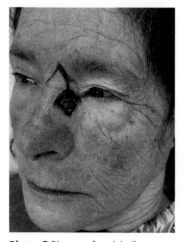 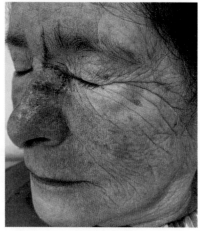

Photo C Planning for glabellar transposition flap in a different patient
Image courtesy of Paul Cherian

Photo D Post repair in the same patient
Image courtesy of Paul Cherian

QUESTION 2
What factors visible in the patient in **Photos A and B** might make you prefer a graft?

Answer
This man has sebaceous skin which has a greater tendency to heal with indented scars, hence minimising the size and number of scars is preferable. He also has rosacea so is at greater risk of red and telangiectatic scars. Lastly, he has very lax medial canthal and eyelid tissue, hence postoperative oedema may take many months to settle.

One should also remain aware of the lacrimal duct and angular blood vessels lateral and deep to this defect, which are at risk when undermining for flap surgery is carried out.

A full-thickness skin graft repair was performed with a preauricular skin donor site that appeared to have a good texture and colour match. The graft was thinned to the mid reticular dermis, fenestrated and secured with 6-0 polyamide. A single basting suture was inserted. A silicone primary dressing and an iodine-based bolus was applied followed by tape. Sutures were removed at 1 week.

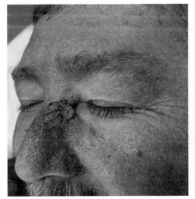

Photo E Post graft repair
Image courtesy of Paul Cherian

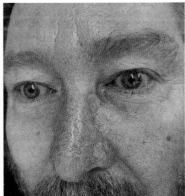

Photo F Result at 2 weeks
Image courtesy of Paul Cherian

QUESTION 3
What can be done to prevent pincushioning of the graft?

Answer

Undermining the edges of the defect, correct sizing (5–10% undersizing) and thinning the graft to sit just below the native skin help with this issue. When suturing, using a "ship-to-shore" with a small bite of the graft and a bigger bite of the defect assist in sitting the graft down into the defect. Fenestration and pexing of the graft allow drainage of oedema and haemoserous fluid, and prevent central festooning. A firm external bolus also prevents fluid build-up. After the graft is well healed and the area is no longer tender (usually a few weeks), firm application of pressure a few times daily with or without Bio-Oil® or other scar treatments appears to hasten resolution of swelling. Take care that any applications are appropriate near the eye.

QUESTION 4
List options for managing pincushioning of the graft.

Answer

- Injected corticosteroids e.g. 0.3–0.8 mL of 5–10 mg/mL triamcinolone acetonide monthly on 2–4 occasions
- Fractionated ablative laser, with or without subcision of the graft and periphery, monthly for 3 sessions; for safety reasons, one would not perform subcision on the eyelid side of the graft
- Ablative laser resurfacing
- Manual or machine-based dermabrasion
- Surgical debulking.

Case 8
Duncan Stanford

A 76-year-old man with two defects after clearance of infiltrative BCCs by Mohs micrographic technique. The size of the defects measured 13 × 16 mm for the left nose bridge and 14 × 18 mm for the right lateral nose (**Photos A** and **B**).

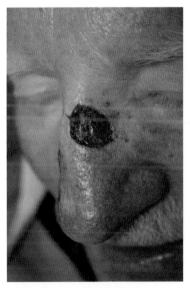

Photo A Left nose bridge defect
Image courtesy of Duncan Stanford

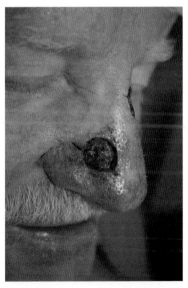

Photo B Right nose sidewall defect
Image courtesy of Duncan Stanford

QUESTION 1

What is your preferred repair option to close the defect in **Photo A** only?

Answer

A glabellar back-cut rotation flap or medially based bilobed transposition flap are simple single-stage repairs with a reliable outcome. Both rely upon recruitment of laxity from the glabellar area; placement of the scar in the natural glabellar lines will be key to obtaining a good result. These repairs will bring the brows closer together—generally not a problem in older individuals. A full-thickness skin graft may provide an excellent outcome in this non-sebaceous upper nasal skin, providing donor skin is chosen carefully. Postauricular skin is often a good texture and colour match; however, the final outcome cannot always be predicted.

Comment on alternatives

An advancement flap with a Burow's triangle or crescent at the alar groove would also work; however, closing the defect across its long axis is usually a less favourable option.

A rhombic transposition flap using the nasal root crease may be possible but would be less reliable and is likely to blunt the natural concavity of the nose bridge. A subcutaneous island pedicle flap from the glabella or lateral nose may have issues in mobilisation due to limited deep tissue beneath the potential flap. Primary closure alone could twist the nose by elevating the contralateral alar rim but may work if combined with second intention healing or a Burow's full-thickness skin graft.

A tunnelled flap or two-stage flap are unnecessarily complex for this shallow medium-sized defect. Second intention healing may result in eyelid distortion, risking an inferior cosmetic result. A split-thickness skin graft should be avoided.

QUESTION 2

What is your preferred repair option to close the defect in **Photo B** only?

Answer

A myocutaneous island pedicle flap (horn variant) or bilobed transposition flap (lateral base) are favoured here.

Comment on alternatives

An advancement flap along the alar crease with perialar crescent or Burow's triangle in the alar groove would work but care must be taken not to depress the alar rim. A back-cut rotation flap tends to move less well than the myocutaneous flap and so may elevate the alar rim. A subcutaneous island pedicle flap might have problems in mobilisation, due to limited deep tissue, resulting in alar elevation. Grafts would be cosmetically inferior in this ruddy sebaceous skin but may be considered in the frail or elderly patient. Second intention healing is likely to elevate the alar rim and should be avoided. Primary closure would result in marked distortion and is not an option. It is too far from the nasofacial junction for a nasolabial transposition flap.

QUESTION 3

What single repair option would close both these defects?

Answer

An advancement flap incorporating both defects into the one closure with medial movement of skin facilitated by removing a Burow's triangle from the alar groove (see **Photo C**).

The elegant design of this single flap allows the joint closure of both defects. The defects are combined by incising from the lower edge of the upper defect across to the upper edge of the lower defect. A second incision from the lower edge of the lower defect extends to the alar groove with removal of a Burow's triangle permitting movement of the nasal skin medially to close both defects (see **Photo D**).

If these defects are closed separately, flap movement must come lateral to or superior to both defects, requiring wider anaesthesia and causing more tissue disturbance.

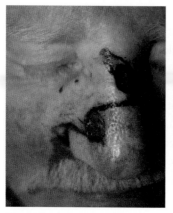

Photo C Advancement flap design with Burow's triangle at the alar groove
Image courtesy of Duncan Stanford

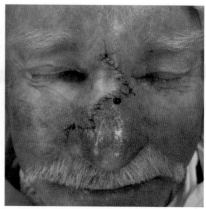

Photo D Advancement flap closure
Image courtesy of Duncan Stanford

QUESTION 4

What is the most striking complication evident in **Photo E**?

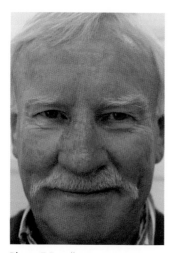

Photo E Excellent outcome at 6 weeks
Image courtesy of Duncan Stanford

Answer

Erythema and telangiectasia—pre-existing nasal telangiectasia and/or rosacea are risk factors for post-surgical exacerbation in all patients.

QUESTION 5

What single treatment would you suggest for the greatest cosmetic improvement?

Answer

Vascular laser (e.g. KTP 532 nm +/− Nd-YAG 1064 nm, pulsed dye 595 nm) or intense pulsed light (IPL).

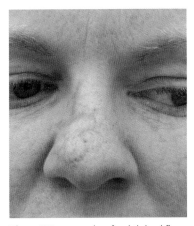

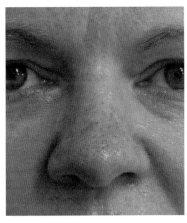

Photo F Two months after bilobed flap repair showing significant telangiectasia
Image courtesy of Shyamala Huilgol

Photo G Excellent outcome following IPL and erbium laser
Image courtesy of Shyamala Huilgol

While both sexes are embarrassed by nasal redness and telangiectasia, men seem more likely to feel that others will think it reflects an alcohol issue and are also unable to resort to cosmetics to hide the problem.

Comment on alternatives

In the absence of any noticeable contour abnormality, standard or fractionated erbium or carbon dioxide lasers won't significantly improve a good-quality scar.

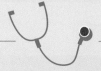

Section 2
Forehead and temple

Case 9
Duncan Stanford

A 64-year-old woman presenting with a recurrent BCC underwent Mohs surgery and had a resultant 14 × 18 mm defect on the right central upper forehead (see **Photo A**).

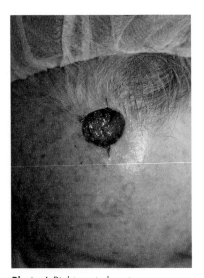

Photo A Right central upper forehead defect

Image courtesy of Duncan Stanford

QUESTION 1

List your three preferred repair options and discuss your reasoning.

Answer

1. Unilateral single-sided advancement/rotation flap
2. Bilateral advancement/rotation flap
3. Bridge (bipedicle) advancement flap

Comment

Sliding (advancement and rotation) flaps are ideal on the forehead to harness the laxity of the lateral forehead and temple, while avoiding elevation of the eyebrows. It is always best to place scar lines in cosmetic junctions and horizontal relaxed skin tension lines or at right angles to these. Given the location of this defect, that means the long flap arm should be placed within or parallel to the hairline or horizontal forehead creases.

It is likely that a unilateral or O–L advancement flap along the hairline would work; the incision could be arced down towards the temple to introduce more rotation if required. In either case, a Burow's triangle or dog ear below the defect will create a vertical scar line. Vertical scars often heal well high on the forehead as the horizontal creases are less prominent here. Vertical scars at any height but within 20 mm of the midline also often do well within the galeal median raphe. (For more inferior defects, a U-plasty advancement flap can shorten the vertical scar by placing more scar lines in horizontal creases.) Better still, with an advancement flap, the horizontal incision could be placed at the inferior edge of the defect with this triangle superior to the defect, above the hairline, so the resultant vertical scar will be concealed by the frontal scalp hair.

If unilateral advancement/rotation flap movement is insufficient, a bilateral or O–T design will mobilise some laxity from the contralateral side. This is preferred when the defect is in the midline.

A bridge or bipedicle flap is another good option here as both scar lines are horizontal and the releasing incision is hidden in the hair. However, it may bring the hairline forward, even if the flap is widely undermined.

Comment on alternatives

Primary repair if oriented horizontally would elevate the right eyebrow and/or pull the hairline forward asymmetrically. A vertical orientation may close large defects in the midline or paramedian forehead but will lead to a larger visible vertical forehead scar and risks dehiscence due to excessive tension and edge necrosis. Second intention healing could work but might elevate the eyebrow. Grafting, while always achievable, would likely lead to an inferior cosmetic result relative to a local flap. A transposition flap would not only be difficult to execute here but would lead to more conspicuous scarring with less favourable diagonal scars. The latter is also true of an island flap regardless of orientation, and the frontalis-based myocutaneous flap design is best reserved for larger, deeper defects, given the risks of greater morbidity.

QUESTION 2

The defect is repaired with a unilateral single-sided advancement flap. Describe the steps in performing this repair, including design, technique, suture materials, dressings and follow-up.

Answer

1. Draw a horizontal line laterally either (a) along the hairline (or just above it) from the superior edge of the defect, or (b) along a horizontal crease from the inferior edge of the defect.

2. Draw a Burow's triangle with base centred on the defect either (a) below the defect or (b) above the defect.

3. Ideally, the horizontal line will be at least one-and-a-half times the length of the vertical line, allowing closure by "rule of halves" principle (L-plasty). However, if there is too much visible puckering of the longer edge, a standing cone needs to be removed at the lateral end of the horizontal excision line and on the opposite side to the flap's Burow's triangle. This will help to equalise the two sides for a superior wound closure. It is often best to plan for this eventuality and anaesthetise appropriately, but only remove this tissue as needed.

4. Incise and undermine the flap in the subcutaneous plane beyond the confines of the planned flap until adequate mobility and tension-free closure is achievable. Undermine the defect edges.

5. After haemostasis is obtained, absorbable buried sutures (e.g. 4-0 or 5-0 poliglecaprone 25 or polyglyconate) are placed to close the defect, with the first key suture closing the primary defect.

6. Insert superficial sutures (e.g. 5-0 or 6-0 nylon or polypropylene) percutaneously (**Photo B**). Alternatively, subcuticular sutures or tissue adhesive may be used.

7. Apply petrolatum and a non-stick dressing followed by a pressure dressing for 48 hours.

8. Verbal and written instructions to patient/carer regarding use of ice packs (hourly for 10–15 minutes on the day of surgery), analgesia (paracetamol as needed), daily wound care (clean with saline or 3% peroxide, apply petrolatum and a non-stick dressing), restricting physical activity, "red flags" (signs of infection, bleeding, flap necrosis, etc.) and contact details.

9. Offer a wound check at about 48 hours to remove pressure dressing or instruct patient to do so and commence daily wound care. Arrange to remove sutures at 7 days and review flap outcomes in about 6–12 weeks. If there has not yet been a general skin check, this could be done at the same time; otherwise, organise this every 6–12 months.

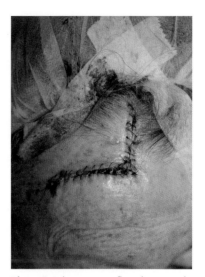

Photo B Advancement flap closure with superior Burow's triangle. Closure was achieved along the horizontal limb by the "rule of halves", with the anticipated Burow's triangle drawn preoperatively not having been required.
Image courtesy of Duncan Stanford

QUESTION 3

List two common *early* side effects specific to this repair at this site that you would warn the patient about.

Answer

1. Postoperative anaesthesia affecting the skin above the horizontal scars — may last for several months. In rare cases, there may be a small area of permanent anaesthesia.

2. Marked bruising and swelling — not uncommon in periorbital area after flap repairs on the forehead. It is helpful to forewarn the patient and reassure them it is temporary but that it may alarm family and friends.

Comment on alternatives

If the flap has been well designed and executed, eyebrow elevation should not occur. Temporary alopecia is quite uncommon in the early postoperative period. (Permanent alopecia a few millimetres wide along the scalp scar line is common but is a long-term complication.) Other risks and complications are less specific to this repair here, but include infection, bleeding, suture reactions, conspicuous scars, etc.

The patient had an excellent long-term outcome (see **Photo C**).

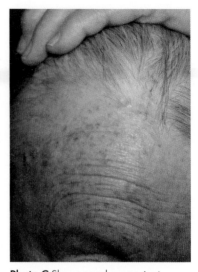

Photo C Shows good cosmesis at 6 weeks due to concealment of scar lines, with further improvement anticipated as scar erythema fades over the next 1–2 months

Image courtesy of Duncan Stanford

Case 10
Richard Turner

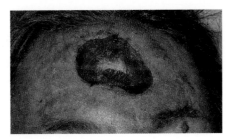

Photo A Post-Mohs defect with central bare bone
Image courtesy of Richard Turner

A 74-year-old woman with a recurrent BCC underwent Mohs surgery, resulting in a central and right lateral forehead defect (**Photo A**) measuring 42 × 62 mm with a central 20 × 20 mm portion of bone denuded of periosteum.

QUESTION 1

What management options exist for exposed bone and what are the consequences of inadequate reconstruction?

Answer

Direct grafting on an avascular bed of this size is not possible. One may carefully chisel or burr off a portion of the outer table of compact bone to expose blood vessels in the underlying spongy bone and thus provide a bed for either immediate split-thickness or delayed split- or full-thickness skin grafting. As bone is insensate, the procedure may be done under local anaesthesia to cover the surrounding tissue but it is most often performed with sedation or general anaesthesia.

Vascularised tissue to cover the bare bone may be provided with local or free flaps. Local flaps can cover small defects. If necessary, the secondary defect or defects created by a larger flap or flaps can be grafted if direct closure is not possible. Galeal flaps may also be harvested from the adjacent scalp to cover the bone and provide a vascularised base for grafting. Free flaps are beyond the remit of this text.

Exposed bone may result from surgery (as in this case), overlying flap or graft failure, drying out of a wound and radiotherapy, resulting in periosteum necrosis and bone desiccation. The resultant wound may take many months to heal or become a permanent ulcer with a significant risk of developing osteomyelitis.

QUESTION 2
What flap reconstructions would you consider and what are their relative merits?

Answer
1. Ipsilateral rotation flap
2. Bilateral advancement flap (modified O–Z)
3. Double rotation (curved O–T) flap
4. Contralateral subgaleal sliding (CLASS) flap[1]

Comment on repairs
This is a complex problem as there is a large facial defect with exposed bone, necessitating vascularised tissue. This cosmetically sensitive area needs good skin matching, restoration of symmetry (level eyebrows) and ensuring that hair-bearing skin is not moved onto the forehead.

An ipsilateral rotation flap would have to be large to cover the area without tension and inevitably will result in significant eyebrow elevation from loss of flap height as it moves into the defect and secondary tissue movement. The orientation of the defect also hinders easy closure by this method. A modified O–Z repair could work with the lower portion of the flap created just above the eyebrow in the horizontal forehead crease and the superior portion following the curving hairline on the contralateral side. A double rotation flap (curved base O–T) could be constructed with enlargement of the defect to the hairline, the upper incision just below the hairline on both sides, possibly with an inferior M-plasty. Standard advancement or rotation flaps with subcutaneous dissection risk flap necrosis due to the high tension needed to close this large defect.

Undermining of the double rotation flap in the subgaleal plane would improve vascularity. The reliable vascularity of the contralateral subgaleal sliding (CLASS) flap[1] was the deciding factor in making our ultimate choice.

QUESTION 3

Describe your design and execution of the CLASS flap. List its advantages and disadvantages.

Answer

1. Mark the flap, extending from the superior defect edge to the contralateral temporal recession, following the frontal hairline. A Burow's triangle is drawn in the temporal scalp recession and used as needed (i.e. creating a Burow's exchange advancement flap) to enhance flap movement.

2. Use supraorbital, supratrochlear and zygomaticofacial nerve blocks with additional infiltration along incision lines for haemostasis. Keeping local anaesthetic volumes low reduces flap bulkiness and enhances closure.

3. Using sterile technique, incise the flap into the subgaleal plane, tying off superficial temporal vessels as needed. Dissect in the relatively bloodless subgaleal plane around the primary and secondary (incision line) defects and then beneath the flap, freeing it from the periosteum of the underlying forehead and extending inferiorly to the supraorbital ridge. If needed, excise and undermine the Burow's triangle. Achieve haemostasis.

4. The key suture closes the defect and is placed from the leading edge of the flap to the lateral (right) defect edge. Place a 4-0 absorbable buried vertical mattress suture to enhance wound edge eversion. Ensure the tension vector is parallel to the ipsilateral eyebrow, keeping the eyebrow as level as possible. Close the remainder of the flap with further buried vertical mattress sutures, spreading the tension evenly along the length of the wound.

5. Excise the inferior standing cone. In this instance, extend into the glabella crease to disguise the incision line.

6. Cutaneous sutures (5-0 nylon or polypropylene) are placed, ensuring good apposition and wound edge eversion (**Photo B**).

Advantages

A very reliable flap as it is broad-based and vascularised from the contralateral superficial temporal, supratrochlear and supraorbital arteries. The skin laxity of the contralateral temple and preauricular skin provides significant movement. The cosmetic outcome is generally good as scars are hidden in the hairline and the colour match is good. The subgaleal dissecting plane preserves function of the temporalis nerve.

Disadvantages

Marked periorbital/facial swelling and bruising is common, with potential for haematoma. Elevation of the contralateral, or even the ipsilateral, eyebrow is possible. The hairline may be altered with advancement of hair-bearing skin onto the forehead without careful flap design. Numbness of the scalp is usual for several months before gradually resolving, but may, on occasion, be permanent.

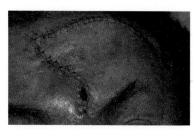

Photo B Post repair, note elevated contralateral eyebrow

Image courtesy of Richard Turner

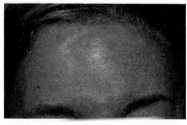

Photo C Three months post surgery with resolved eyebrow elevation

Image courtesy of Richard Turner

Comment

Note the mild left eyebrow elevation in the preclosure image (**Photo A**) and some enhancement postoperatively (**Photo B**). This had improved at 1 week and returned to normal at 3 months (**Photo C**). Pre- and postoperative photography is important in documenting any natural asymmetry.

Reference

1. Hussain W. The contralateral subgaleal sliding flap for the single stage reconstruction of large defects of the temple and lateral forehead. Br J Dermatol 2014; 170: 952–5.

Case 11
Tim Rutherford and Shyamala Huilgol

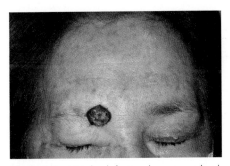

Photo A Post-Mohs defect and previous island pedicle flap scar lines

Image courtesy of Tim Rutherford

A 61-year-old woman had Mohs surgery for a recurrent micronodular BCC on the right medial eyebrow (**Photo A**). A previous island pedicle flap had resulted in sparse eyebrow hair and scarring. The Mohs surgery defect measured 15 × 17 mm.

QUESTION 1
List your three preferred repair options, and include your reasoning.

Answer

1. Laterally based island pedicle flap. The medial eyebrow is of greater cosmetic importance than the lateral eyebrow, so advancing the remaining (even sparse) eyebrow medially produces superior results compared to retaining the lateral brow at the expense of the medial eyebrow. Island pedicle flaps are reliable where previous scarring exists, particularly where the pedicle includes muscle, as in this case.

2. O–T or H-type advancement flaps. These flaps would satisfactorily transfer the remaining lateral eyebrow medially, but scarring from previous surgery, coupled with purely cutaneous pedicles, gives a greater risk of flap necrosis. H-type flaps may result in puckering and dog ears unless Burow's triangles are removed.

3. Hair-bearing full-thickness skin graft. This is the least preferred repair due to unpredictability of skin/hair match and take. In male patients, the sideburn can be a suitable donor site for total or near total eyebrow loss, but attention must be paid to matching hair shaft direction and counselling patients about the longer growth phase with the resultant need for regular trimming.

Comment on alternatives

Primary closure and other local flaps would fail in re-creating the important medial brow and might distort the residual brow and upper eyelid.

QUESTION 2

You elect to use a lenticular island pedicle flap. Describe your design considerations.

Answer

The lenticular island pedicle flap is a modification of the traditional triangular island pedicle flap that incorporates a rotational element. By doing so, it avoids the triangular scar lines that, in this case, would produce a prominent vertical suture line at the advancing edge of the flap. The lenticular flap width should be approximately the diameter of the surgical defect, with a flap length 2–3 times the diameter of the defect. The rotational element should conform to the natural curve of the lateral eyebrow. A small triangle should be excised from the opposite side of the defect to alter the defect shape to a "teardrop" and better accommodate the flap tip, thus avoiding scar lines perpendicular to the relaxed skin tension lines and resulting in an aesthetically superior scar (**Photo B and C**).

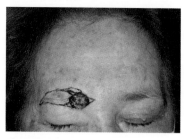

Photo B Design of lenticular flap
Image courtesy of Tim Rutherford

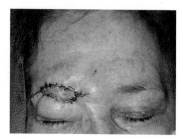

Photo C Flap closure
Image courtesy of Tim Rutherford

QUESTION 3

The patient contacts you 6 days later complaining of "significant bruising" **(Photo D)**. What is your management?

Answer

Assess for haematoma and infection: a detailed history including onset and progression, postoperative blood loss, pain and discharge. Review general health and medications (see next question). Make a visual inspection and palpate the surgical site.

Once a simple ecchymosis is confirmed, reassurance and education are usually all that is required. The bruising should move down the cheek and fade over 1–2 weeks. Cosmetic camouflage can be used but makeup should be avoided over the wound until sutures are removed and suture holes have re-epithelialised.

If desired, consider hastening the resolution of bruising with heparinoid cream 2–4 times daily, or the use of pulsed dye or potassium titanyl phosphate (KTP) lasers (with an eye shield if treating within the orbital rim). At 6 days post surgery, ice packs, compression and avoidance of exertion are unlikely to help, being most important in the first 48 hours.

Document your findings and advice provided, take clinical photographs and arrange regular reviews until resolution.

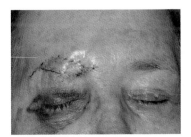

Photo D Results at 6 days postoperatively with significant bruising
Image courtesy of Tim Rutherford

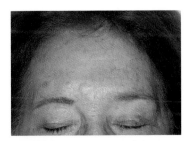

Photo E Results at 10 months. Excellent recreation of brow, supplemented by eyebrow pencil
Image courtesy of Tim Rutherford

QUESTION 4

What factors may have contributed to the prominent bruising?

Answer

Patient factors include coagulopathies, underlying systemic disease (e.g. liver and kidney failure, haematologic disorders), alcohol consumption and medication, both prescribed and over the counter, including herbal supplements. Older patients with atrophic and fragile skin have a higher likelihood of bruising. Certain nutritional deficiencies increase the risk of bruising, as does non-adherence to postoperative advice and restrictions.

Surgical factors. Bruising is increased with prominent perioperative bleeding. Factors include inadequate haemostasis, increased cutaneous blood flow due to rosacea, where surgery involves underlying skeletal muscle or arteries, when wide undermining is performed and in certain higher risk sites—particularly periorbital, perioral and periauricular. Where the risk of haematoma and bruising is considered high, a drain and/or compression dressings may be used.

Some bruising is normal, however, and should be emphasised when obtaining informed consent. Use clear language—that is, "black eye"—so that patients can avoid social engagements for the expected natural resolution period of 10–14 days.

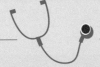

Section 3

Perioral

Case 12
Duncan Stanford

A 70-year-old woman presented with a recurrent nodular BCC in the apical triangle of the left upper lip after serial curettage and electrosurgery two years prior. The BCC was cleared by Mohs micrographic surgery in two stages, leaving a defect of 18 × 20 mm (**Photo A**).

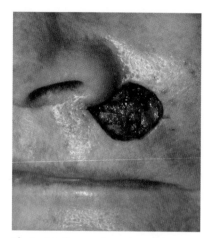

Photo A Left upper lip and medial cheek defect

Image courtesy of Duncan Stanford

QUESTION 1

List your three preferred repair options and discuss your reasoning.

Answer

1. Subcutaneous island pedicle flap—ideal as it places two of the three scar lines in cosmetic junctions.

   For a larger/deeper defect, a tunnelled variant from the medial cheek can be transposed into the defect without transgressing the melolabial fold.

2. Rotation flap—upper limb extending laterally along the melolabial fold; inferior dog ear placed in perioral rhytides and with M-plasty to avoid crossing vermilion-cutaneous junction.

   For larger defects and those extending further down the cutaneous lip cosmetic unit, a rotation flap can be combined with an inferior wedge resection to reduce the defect size.

3. Banner transposition flap—There are two possible designs recruiting medial cheek laxity. The preferred option is an inferiorly based transposition flap from nasofacial sulcus with the pivot point redundancy removed from the upper nasolabial fold. The alternative design is a superiorly based flap from the nasolabial fold with the rotation pucker in the alar groove. This flap design needs significantly more rotation and cheek advancement.

   Both flaps have the disadvantage of crossing, and therefore blunting, the upper melolabial fold and they are also prone to trapdooring. The superiorly based design will be more affected by trapdooring due to inability to drain tissue fluid inferiorly.

Comment on alternatives

This defect is too large for a perialar crescentic side-to-side repair alone, although this repair could achieve partial closure allowing second intention healing of a residual central defect in the alar groove. A wedge resection alone here is not appropriate, but it could reduce a larger, more inferiorly extending defect in combination with a rotation or cheek advancement flap repair. It is too lateral for a crescentic advancement flap. It is too large for an O–T advancement flap with its base in the nasal sill and alar groove, as it would pull the philtrum laterally leading to asymmetry. A full-thickness skin graft is reasonable with careful donor site selection (medial cheek) but is unlikely to achieve cosmesis comparable to a well-executed flap. Split-thickness skin grafts are contraindicated with poor cosmetic outcomes. Interpolation flaps are unnecessarily complex and inconvenient here (they may have a role in a more significant defect in a patient with high cosmetic expectations, in which case referral for plastics reconstruction should be considered).

QUESTION 2

The defect was repaired with a subcutaneous island pedicle flap. Describe the steps in design and execution of this flap.

Answer

1. Outline the triangular flap with the lateral long arm in the nasolabial fold and the medial arm from the lower medial defect edge to the lower nasolabial fold. The leading edge corresponds to the base of the triangle, which advances V–Y to the alar groove.

2. Use an infraorbital nerve block, then local anaesthetic infiltration.

3. Using sterile technique, incise the flap to the deep subcutaneous tissue. Avoid extending too deeply (i.e. into underlying muscle) as this risks motor nerve damage.

4. Undermine around the flap in the subcutaneous plane using surgical scissors perpendicular to the incision lines to tease open the space between the fatty pedicle and surrounding skin. Avoid compromising the pedicle's blood supply.

5. Undermine the leading flap edge in the upper subcutis and the flap tail in the deep subcutis to leave a central monopedicle approximately one-third of the flap length.

6. Using a skin hook, advance the leading edge to check for adequate flap movement and ascertain where there are areas of tension. If required, cautiously insert the scissors vertically into the sides of the pedicle and bluntly dissect to loosen the pedicle further while leaving the vessels and nerves intact, until the flap closes the defect without tension.

7. Place the first buried absorbable suture (e.g. 5-0 poliglecaprone 25) from the underside of the undermined advancing portion of the flap (a few millimetres behind the leading edge) to the base of the defect. This pulls the flap down into the defect, producing visible depression, and reduces the risk of trapdooring. The second buried suture should pull the leading edge of the flap across the defect to close it, then a third buried suture is placed behind the tail to close the secondary defect. Other buried sutures are placed around the flap perimeter as required.

8. Insert a few interrupted cutaneous non-absorbable sutures (e.g. 5-0 or 6-0 nylon), including a tip-stitch to position the tail correctly, then close with running sutures. Ensure that the tail is flush with the surrounding skin (**Photo B**).

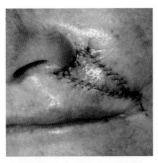

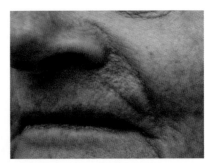

Photo B Subcutaneous island pedicle flap repair
Image courtesy of Duncan Stanford

Photo C Outcome at 2 months
Image courtesy of Duncan Stanford

QUESTION 3

What complication common to this repair is evident in **Photo C** and what treatment options will you discuss with the patient?

Answer

Pincushioning or trapdoor effect—due to flap oedema and circumferential scar contraction.

1. Observation—may improve a little over time; may not concern this patient (**Photo D**).
2. Intralesional corticosteroid—triamcinolone acetonide 10 mg/mL (Kenacort A10®) 0.4–0.8 mL into the subcutis of the mid-flap pincushioned area until evenly blanched and oedematous; may need to be repeated in 4–6 weeks.
3. Fractionated ablative (or less effective option of non-ablative) laser, possibly in combination with subcision, is effective in reducing the scar troughing.
4. Surgical flap revision—in more severe or unresponsive cases.

Comment on alternatives

Traditional laser resurfacing is likely to lead to long-term hypopigmentation in the area.

QUESTION 4

What steps can be taken in executing this flap to minimise the risk of pincushioning?

Answer

1. Slight undersizing of the flap to place it on the stretch
2. Increasing the depth of the defect slightly to ensure that the flap can sit down within it
3. Undermining defect edges to reduce tethering, produce a more horizontal scar and lessen the tendency to scar inversion
4. Pexing sutures from the underside of the flap to the base of the defect to produce slight central concavity of the flap
5. Placing buried sutures to produce central concavity and stretch of the flap

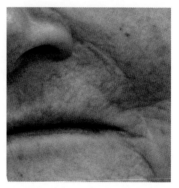

Photo D Result at 2 years. Note re-creation of the nasolabial fold in original position through upper flap and persistence of some inferior flap fullness

Image courtesy of Duncan Stanford

6. Placing percutaneous sutures from "ship-to-shore", taking small, more superficial bites of the flap and larger, slightly deeper bites of the surrounding skin to recess the flap

Case 13
Niamh O'Sullivan and Shyamala Huilgol

A 69-year-old woman presented with a combined cutaneous upper lip and vermilion defect measuring 11 × 14 mm following Mohs surgery to a superficially invasive, well-differentiated squamous cell carcinoma (**Photo A**). A previous wedge excision to the right central upper lip had flattened this philtral column and obliterated the Cupid's bow.

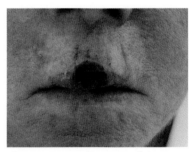

Photo A Post-Mohs surgery defect
Image courtesy of Shyamala Huilgol

QUESTION 1
What are your three favoured repair options? Comment on their relative merits.

Answer
1. Double island pedicle (V–Y) flaps — cutaneous and mucosal
2. Full-thickness graft to cutaneous lip and mucosal flap
3. Wedge repair

Comment
The two very different subunits of cutaneous and mucosal lip must be repaired with matching tissue. It is also important to respect the philtral columns as subunit boundaries, to try and re-create the Cupid's bow and avoid effacement of the white roll. In older patients, these boundaries are often less distinct and therefore less important.

Function is also essential, with the orbicularis oris being vital in speech, whistling, kissing and creation of a seal for eating and drinking.

The *cutaneous defect* may be repaired with a superiorly based V–Y flap, O–U advancement flap along the philtral columns with Burow's triangles under the nasal sill or with a full-thickness graft. Shaping of the lower margin of the cutaneous flap can re-create the Cupid's bow. If grafting, it may be best to widen the defect to align with the philtral columns and consider enlarging it vertically to encompass the entire philtral subunit.

The *vermilion defect* may be repaired with a V–Y flap from the inner mucosal lip, a double rotation flap along the vermilion border or a mucosal advancement flap with excision of the residual exposed vermilion.

Using two different repairs is more complex and requires greater experience to get a good outcome. The combination of double V–Y flaps preserves lip width and may obtain excellent cosmesis and function[1]. The Cupid's bow is very challenging to re-create and often falls short of the desired outcome. When closing repairs along the vermilion border, it is often difficult to re-create the white roll that lies immediately superior. Grafts are prone to difficulties in obtaining initial take and long-term colour and contour match. (Hair-bearing donor skin must be used in males.) Mucosal tissue is often pinker than the native vermilion and may be prone to ongoing peeling. Excision of the entire upper vermilion may result in permanent dysaesthesia.

Primary closure with a wedge is the simplest and most reliable repair but will obliterate midline structures: the Cupid's bow, philtrum and philtral crests, and possibly the frenulum. When closing the two peaks of the Cupid's bow to each other, a central upward tenting or trigone deformity of the lip may result **(Photo B)**. The lip width will be reduced and the strength and function of orbicularis oris may be compromised if not adequately repaired. Prolonged dysaesthesia may occur.

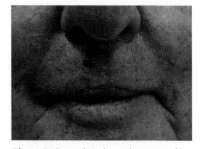

Photo B Central V-shaped tenting of lip following wedge repair of Cupid's bow defect in a different patient
Image courtesy of Shyamala Huilgol

Comment on alternatives

Flaps recruiting lateral lip skin such as V–Y flaps with both cutaneous and vermilion components or advancement flaps along the nasal sill and vermilion border will cross the philtral columns and efface these and the Cupid's bow. Second intention healing could be used for the vermilion defect and may be hastened with biologic wound dressings such as acellular dermal matrices. Disadvantages include cosmesis and wound care while healing, possible infection, dietary restrictions and the risk of visible and symptomatic hypertrophic scarring. Mucosal grafts may be difficult to match; the dynamic nature of this area complicates dressing and wound care and may impact upon graft survival. The "Frogger flap" is a novel but complex quadruple rhomboid flap which preserves aesthetic subunits in combined cutaneous and vermilion central upper lip defects.[2]

QUESTION 2

Describe the design and execution of double island pedicle flaps in this defect.

Answer

1. Design and mark the flaps and the vermilion border with a surgical marker. The superior flap triangle should follow the philtral columns superiorly and may extend upwards into the nasal columella. The inferior flap triangle may be extended to the gingival sulcus if needed (**Photo C**).
2. Perform bilateral infra-orbital blocks, then infiltrate additional local anaesthesia with adrenaline for haemostasis and stabilisation of the lip.
3. Use sterile technique.
4. Mark the vermilion border with light scoring or sutures.
5. Incise the flaps down to muscle, then undermine the leading edge of the flaps and lateral edges of the defect. Free the flap's tail at its depth. Mobilise both flaps.

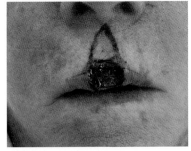

Photo C Design of the double V–Y flaps with Cupid's bow drawn on cutaneous flap

Image courtesy of Shyamala Huilgol

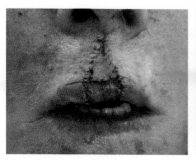

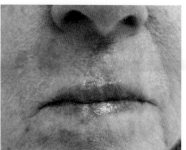

Photo D Flap repair with reconstruction of Cupid's bow
Image courtesy of Shyamala Huilgol

Photo E Good outcome at 3 months. Note slight pinkness of mucosal flap
Image courtesy of Shyamala Huilgol

6. The key suture in both flaps is a buried 5-0 absorbable suture from the leading undersurface of the flap (approximately 5 mm back from the advancing edge) to the depth of the defect.

7. Close the cutaneous defect first and accurately align at the vermilion border, then close the mucosal defect with its flap, allowing some central excess tissue in both flaps to re-create the Cupid's bow later.

8. Use interrupted 6-0 nylon cutaneous sutures to reinforce correct positioning at the vermilion border. Absorbable 5-0 or 6-0 glycolide L-lactide or catgut sutures are used on the mucosa.

9. Use buried and then running sutures to close the secondary defects and then the flaps.

10. After satisfactory placement of both flaps, trim the advancing edges to re-create the Cupid's bow and place cutaneous sutures (**Photo D**). Late review of the outcome should be arranged (**Photo E**).

QUESTION 3
What can be done to increase flap mobilisation?

Answer
*   Ensure adequate undermining of the leading edges of the flaps and release of the tails.
*   Insert a skin hook at the leading edge of the flap, gently slide it forward and then release any tethering.
*   Ask the patient to animate, watch for points of tethering and release these.

- Undermine both primary and secondary defects.
- After placing key sutures, close the secondary defects next.
- Consider very careful undermining of the lateral flap edges.

QUESTION 4

This patient has a history of MRSA and poor dentition. What can be done pre- and postoperatively to help minimise the risk of infection?

Answer

Preop:
- Dental and hygienist review for meticulous cleaning of dentures or devices.
- Twice daily flossing and 0.2% chlorhexidine mouth wash.
- Decolonisation for 5 days with intranasal 2% mupirocin nasal ointment twice daily combined with daily 2% chlorhexidine gluconate or 1% triclosan body wash. Family members may also decolonise.
- Antibiotics—seek microbiology advice with results of previous microbiology results and consult local infection protocols. Typical regimes use trimethoprim/sulfamethoxazole or clindamycin.

Postop:
- Saline mouth washes (½ tsp salt in 250 mL of warm water) after meals.
- 0.2% chlorhexidine mouth wash, three times daily until suture removal.
- Mupirocin 2% ointment to suture line, twice daily until suture removal.

References
1. Huilgol SC, Ma JH, Hills RJ. Double island pedicle or V-Y flap repair for partial-thickness combined defects of the cutaneous and mucosal lip. J Am Acad Dermatol 2014 Dec; 71(6): 1198–1203.
2. Robinson JN, Elhage SA, Marturano MN, Teng E. The "Frogger flap": A novel quadruple rhomboid flap for complex central upper lip reconstruction. Plastic and Reconstructive Surgery. Global Open 2022 Feb; 10(2): e4072.

Case 14
Niamh O'Sullivan and Shyamala Huilgol

A 54-year-old woman underwent Mohs surgery for a thinly invasive, well-differentiated SCC on the right lower lip with a final tumour-free defect measuring 14 × 9 mm (**Photo A**).

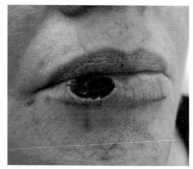

Photo A Post-Mohs surgery vermilion defect

Image courtesy of Shyamala Huilgol

QUESTION 1

List your five favoured repair options. Comment on their relative advantages and disadvantages.

Answer

1. Wedge resection
2. Mucosal advancement flap
3. Bilateral vermilion rotation flap
4. V–Y mucosal advancement flap
5. Second intention healing

Comment

Full-thickness wedge resections may be used for defects up to 30% of the lower lip without significant microstomia. This repair is robust and relatively straightforward. The orbicularis oris must be adequately repaired with layered suturing to prevent issues with oral competence, including speech, dribbling and whistling. The reduced lip width may affect denture insertion; denture use should be assessed beforehand, especially before larger resections. The two sides of the lip must be perfectly aligned, particularly the vermilion border but also the wet line. Vermilion border mismatch is problematic if it occurs and is more obvious in the younger patient. The most difficult wedge reconstructions are in the lateral lip where there are significant differences in the height and depth of the vermilion on either side. Reconstructions in which the border alignment is prioritised at the expense of the wet line may result in the wet line step off, fat lip and trigone deformities. The repair extends into the adjacent lower cutaneous lip and chin units with more sebaceous skin and a tendency to indented scarring. One should avoid crossing the central prominent mental crease with T- or M-plasty variations to the lower end of the wedge. Temporary dysaesthesia is common, but most recover normal sensation over some months.

Advancement of the labial mucosa is a simple and robust repair which maintains the lip width. It is best in shallow defects where most, if not all, the muscle has been preserved. Reported techniques vary greatly in the amount of suggested submucosal undermining—from none to extending all the way to the gingival sulcus—without apparent alteration in cosmetic outcomes. The scar is well hidden along the cosmetic unit junction but may be noticeable when stretched with a wide smile. An added benefit is the removal of surrounding actinically damaged mucosa, which might otherwise require treatment with a laser vermilionectomy or topical 5-fluorouracil. Significant and permanent dysaesthesia occurs in up to 30% of cases and may reflect mental nerve damage during undermining. Exteriorisation of the wet mucosa results in a redder lip which may also remain dry and peel. The lip is usually somewhat flatter with loss of the white roll. In males, the secondary movement of lower lip skin may pull coarse hair-bearing skin inwards with bothersome bristling of the hairs against the upper lip and minor difficulties when shaving near the altered vermilion border.

Bilateral vermilion rotation and *V–Y mucosal flaps* both confine the scar to the vermilion, maintain lip contour and width, avoid unnecessary resection of orbicularis oris muscle and minimise dysaesthesia associated with mucosal advancement flaps. The bilateral rotation flap is best suited to smaller, centrally located defects, but may be modified and used in this lateral defect. Secondary movement of the cutaneous lip inwards with the rotation flap may have similar issues as described for the mucosal advancement flap. The V–Y may be used anywhere along the lower lip. This flap may be slightly depressed and have a noticeably darker pink hue, dryness and peeling.

Second intention healing[1] avoids further surgery and the attendant risks of pain, bleeding, haematoma, dysaesthesia, suture reactions, dehiscence and flap necrosis. Excellent cosmetic results may be achieved. The disadvantage is extended healing with more difficult wound care and an increased risk of infection. Antiviral prophylaxis may be used in those with a personal or partner history of herpes labialis. Acellular dermal matrices may expedite healing.

Comment on alternative

Mucosal grafts are difficult to immobilise in this site.

QUESTION 2

The patient wanted Mohs surgery but described herself as "terrified of needles". How can you reduce anxiety for local anaesthesia procedures?

Answer

- Preoperative patient education, both written and verbal, preferably with a family member present.
- Clear, consistent and kind communication from the surgeon and team at all times.
- Calm and professional surroundings with soothing music and a blanket, warmed if possible.
- Anxiolytics—a number of different benzodiazepines and even clonidine may be used. The authors use alprazolam 0.5 mg (0.25 mg in the elderly) one hour preoperatively with additional doses as required or lorazepam 2 mg the night before and 1 mg on the morning of surgery. All patients having anxiolytics require an escort and for the first 24 hours postoperatively. Check that the preoperative blood pressure is normal, exclude orthostatic hypotension and liaise with the patient's general practitioner regarding general health and mental state before prescribing these agents.

- The risks of benzodiazepines include oversedation, respiratory depression, unsteadiness, confusion, disinhibition and patient amnesia regarding consent and discussion of repair options.

QUESTION 3
How can you reduce the pain from local anaesthesia in this area?

Answer
- Topical anaesthesia to the mucosa for 1–3 minutes: dry mucosa with gauze, then apply either 20% benzocaine or 5% lignocaine gel with a cotton tip, or use a dental roll/pledget soaked in 1–2% lignocaine.
- Intraoral (rather than percutaneous) mental nerve blocks.
- Ropivacaine (0.75% +/− adrenaline) or lignocaine buffered with 8.4% sodium bicarbonate to reduce stinging.
- Fine needles (27–30G) with Luer lock or dental syringes.
- Slow injection technique.
- Distraction techniques, including music, soothing conversation, handholding, stress balls, vibrating devices or tapping.

QUESTION 4
How would you perform an intraoral mental nerve block?

Answer
1. Position the patient flat with the head and neck supported and level with your elbows.
2. Use protective eyewear and non-sterile gloves.
3. Using the above measures to reduce pain, hold the lower lip between thumb and index finger and retract the lower lip, placing the fourth finger below the mental foramen.
4. Inject in the gingival sulcus between and parallel to the premolars, to 10 mm depth and without touching the bone. Withdraw immediately if there is paraesthesia, as this may indicate intra-foraminal injection. Aspirate to exclude intravascular injection, then inject 1–3 mL of local anaesthetic. Massage externally for 10 seconds. Wait for at least 10 minutes.

QUESTION 5

A wedge resection was chosen to reconstruct this defect. How can you avoid vermilion border misalignment?

Answer

- Mark the vermilion border with a surgical marker pre-anaesthetic. After anaesthesia, use a 5-0 silk suture, light scoring with scalpel blade or temporary tattoo with methylene blue on a 27G needle.
- Use blocks to reduce local anaesthesia infiltration, distortion and adrenaline-induced blanching.
- Careful reapproximation of all layers of the repair (**Photos B** and **C**).
- Manage unequal lip widths either by cutting diagonally across the lateral margin to increase its cross-sectional width or by aligning the wet line first and then using sliding Z-plasties to realign the vermilion.[2]

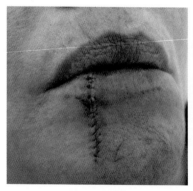
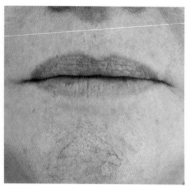

Photo B Immediate post reconstruction demonstrating excellent apposition of tissue and vermilion alignment
Image courtesy of Shyamala Huilgol

Photo C Excellent outcome at 9 months post surgery
Image courtesy of Shyamala Huilgol

References

1. Leonard AL, Hanke CW. Second intention healing for intermediate and large postsurgical defects of the lip. J Am Acad Dermatol 2007; 57: 832–835.
2. Wentzell J, Lund J. Z-plasty innovations in vertical lip reconstructions. Dermatol Surg 2011; 37(11): 1646–1662.

Case 15
Karyn Lun and Shyamala Huilgol

A 54-year-old woman underwent Mohs surgery to a poorly defined nodular and superficial BCC on the right chin with the final tumour-free defect measuring 10 × 13 mm (**Photo A**).

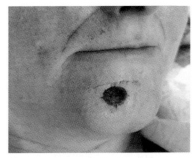

Photo A Post-Mohs surgery defect on chin with mental crease marked pre-operatively
Image courtesy of Shyamala Huilgol

QUESTION 1
List three closure options for this defect and comment on their relative merits.

Answer
1. Unilateral or bilateral rotation flap
2. Subcutaneous island pedicle flap
3. Rhombic transposition flap

Comment
There is not much tissue laxity in this area due to underlying mentalis muscle insertion and the bony prominence. Thicker, sebaceous skin on the chin is more prone to poor scarring; careful planning and execution is also necessary to ensure all dog ears lie flat in this more difficult skin. Many patients have existing telangiectasia, which are increased post surgery

around the scars, making them more obvious. If possible, it is best not to cross the jawline as indented scarring may result.

A unilateral or bilateral rotation flap could be designed with the arc of the flap along the mental crease (**Photo B**). An island pedicle flap with one long arm along the mental crease would hide one of the scars while displacing any downwards pull on the lower lip laterally and spreading it across the length of the flap. A superiorly based rhombic transposition flap could move tissue from the central lower chin but would create more obvious geometrical scarring in the centre of the subunit. It is also prone to trapdooring, especially when superiorly based. (An inferiorly based flap is a poor option as it would cross the mental crease.)

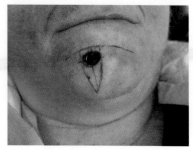

Photo B Double rotation flap plan. Note enlargement of defect to reach the more favourable mental crease
Image courtesy of Shyamala Huilgol

Comment on alternatives

Primary closure is less desirable as horizontal orientation may result in eclabium, while vertical orientation would cross the mental crease. Second intention healing has potential for eclabium and noticeable distortion of the mental crease. A graft would give a poor cosmetic outcome in this sebaceous skin.

QUESTION 2

A bilateral rotation flap was performed (**Photo C**). The patient returned for review at day 4 post surgery (**Photo D**). What has occurred?

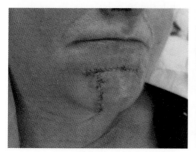

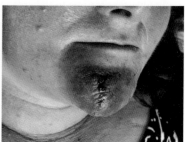

Photo C Post-flap closure
Image courtesy of Shyamala Huilgol

Photo D Day 4 post Mohs surgery
Image courtesy of Shyamala Huilgol

Answer

There is marked discoloration and palpable swelling, indicating a postoperative haematoma. There is some ooze, suggesting that there may be active bleeding.

QUESTION 3

Why may this problem have occurred?

Answer

- On the chin, the mentalis muscle insertion into the dermis predisposes to bleeding and increases the risk of marked bruising and haematoma. It is important to discuss this preoperatively.
- Surgical technique—insufficient haemostasis, unrecognised vessel damage at time of closure.
- Underlying patient factors such as anticoagulation, haematological abnormality, major medical illnesses such as hepatic or renal failure, untreated or poorly controlled hypertension. These are usually identified at the preoperative consultation.
- Postoperative infection.

- Failure to carry out postoperative recommendations for hourly ice packs, avoidance of facial movement (including excessive chewing and talking) on the day of surgery and avoidance of exercise and other exertion until suture removal.
- Inadvertent trauma to the area (e.g. children or pets).

QUESTION 4
Outline your management options.

Answer

1. Assess the situation. Ask whether there has been ongoing blood loss or pain. Review medical history and assess for a coagulopathy.
2. Discuss the situation and treatment options with the patient.
3. Commence appropriate broad-spectrum oral antibiotic (e.g. cephalexin 500 mg tds or qid for 5–7 days).
4. If there has been no recent blood loss, palpate to see if the swelling is fluctuant:
    a. If so, percutaneous evacuation may be attempted:
        i. with appropriate consent, positioning and preparation
        ii. infiltrate 1% lignocaine with 1:200,000 adrenaline
        iii. insert a sharp 18G needle with 5 mL Luer lock syringe attached and attempt aspiration
    b. If this fails, one may also open a small length of the wound (e.g. 10 mm) and attempt expression of the haematoma.
5. In the presence of ongoing blood loss, perform open evacuation:
    a. carefully remove all cutaneous and buried sutures, completely open the flap and remove the haematoma. Saline-soaked gauze may be helpful to gently remove the clotted blood as it is often adherent to the tissues.
    b. achieve haemostasis with electrosurgery. There may be one obvious source or there may be generalised ooze from the mentalis muscle.
    c. re-suture the flap with buried then cutaneous sutures.
    d. in the presence of ongoing mild bleeding, consider adding tranexamic acid 500–1000 mg bd–tds for 3–5 days and placing a drain. Tranexamic acid is renally excreted and the dose should be

reduced in renal impairment. If more marked bleeding persists, seek haematologist advice.

e. give detailed verbal and printed postoperative instructions regarding ice packs and rest.

f. explain the expected clinical course for marked bruising and colour progression from purple to green to yellow with gradual extension from the chin to the neck and even the upper chest, with resolution taking 2–3 weeks.

g. review at 1–3 days for a wound check, then consider permitting the patient to carry out daily wound care.

h. removal of sutures at 7 days (**Photo E**).

6. Observation and supportive measures only

a. later presentation (14 days or more) with non-fluctuant swelling indicates the haematoma is organising and unsuitable for evacuation

b. explain that resolution may take several weeks, with significant temporary induration

c. commence appropriate broad-spectrum antibiotic

d. organise regular postoperative reviews

e. advise to commence massage at least 1 week post removal of sutures.

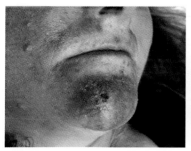
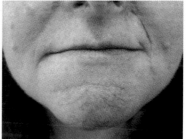

Photo E Note persistent erythema, discolouration and minor crusting at 1 week
Image courtesy of Shyamala Huilgol

Photo F Good surgical result at 3 months, with the primary scar line along the mental crease. Note enhancement of preexisting telangiectasia which may be treated with vascular laser or intense pulsed light
Image courtesy of Shyamala Huilgol

Section 4
Cheeks

Case 16
Karyn Lun and Shyamala Huilgol

Consider these three moderate to large medial cheek defects (**Photos A, B and C**).

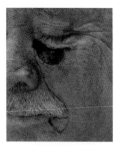

Photo A Moderate
30 × 15 mm defect in
64-year-old man
Image courtesy of Shyamala
Huilgol

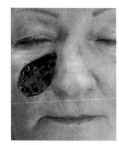

Photo B Large 47 ×
27 mm defect in
51-year-old woman
Image courtesy of
Shyamala Huilgol

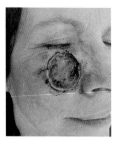

Photo C Large 28
× 32 mm defect in
60-year-old woman.
Note planned minor
re-excision of margins,
drawn in purple, which
will further enlarge the
defect.
Image courtesy of
Shyamala Huilgol

QUESTION 1
List three flap closure options for this medial cheek location.

Answer
1. Unilateral cheek advancement flap with Burow's triangle
2. Subcutaneous island pedicle flap +/− lenticular variant
3. Mustarde cheek rotation flap

QUESTION 2

Discuss the relative advantages and disadvantages of these closures for this site.

Answer

- Unilateral cheek advancement flap with Burow's triangle:
  - best for small to moderate defects that are bigger horizontally than vertically, and for those at or close to the nasofacial sulcus
  - scar lines well hidden in infra-orbital crease, nasofacial sulcus, nasolabial fold and infra-oral crease or marionette line
  - small risk of lower eyelid oedema due to disrupted lymphatic drainage
  - risk of ectropion—pexing suture must be used.
- Subcutaneous island pedicle flap:
  - best for small to moderate defects at or close to the nasofacial sulcus
  - classic design best for defects that are larger horizontally than vertically, but consider "Pac-man" and lenticular variants for larger defects and those with less favourable geometry
  - medial scar line hidden in nasofacial sulcus and nasolabial fold, but lateral scar line visible and may indent, given the sebaceous nature of cheek skin
  - often pincushions
  - higher risk of ectropion with classic flap design due to tension vectors and more difficult flap mobilisation compared to the other two flaps—pexing sutures essential.
- Mustarde cheek rotation flap:
  - reliable repair for medium to large medial cheek defects. May be used away from the nasofacial sulcus, but this placement gives the best cosmesis
  - scar lines lie largely in cosmetic unit junctions—nasofacial sulcus, nasolabial fold, infra-orbital crease and preauricular crease
  - requires significant amounts of local anaesthetic—injections may be poorly tolerated and some risk of local anaesthetic toxicity
  - medial displacement of beard/sideburn

- early lower eyelid oedema common due to disruption of lymphatic drainage
- risk of ectropion—pexing sutures required.

QUESTION 3

Describe how you would perform a unilateral cheek advancement flap with Burow's triangle for **Photo A,** including site-specific considerations.

Answer

1. Design: follow the nasofacial sulcus and nasolabial fold downwards. Plan the superior dog ear either in the infra-orbital crease or pointing diagonally down and across the medial cheek. Place a generous Burow's triangle beneath the oral commissure, in the infra-orbital crease (**Photo D**).

2. Use an infra-orbital nerve block, wait for some minutes, then infiltrate the entire flap and surrounds.

3. Using sterile technique, incise the vertical line and excise the Burow's triangle (but not the superior dog ear), then undermine the flap in the mid-high subcutaneous plane. Obtain haemostasis.

4. Place a 4-0 or 5-0 absorbable pexing suture from the flap's undersurface and a few mm back from the leading edge to the infraorbital maxilla. This should close the defect without tension and remove any drag on the lower eyelid. A noticeable dimple is often seen; this will resolve over a few months.

5. Close the Burow's triangle, then along the nasofacial sulcus, with 5-0 buried absorbable sutures, deliberately lifting the flap upwards.

6. Excise the superior dog ear, trying to place it within the infra-orbital crease. If this will pull on the eyelid, consider angling it down and laterally across the upper medial cheek. Place cutaneous sutures with good apposition (**Photo E**).

7. Give written and verbal postoperative instructions. Arrange removal of sutures at 1 week and longer-term review at 3 months (**Photo F**).

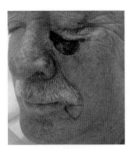

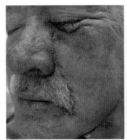

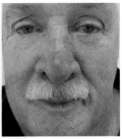

Photo D Advancement flap plan with Burow's triangle
Image courtesy of Shyamala Huilgol

Photo E Post repair. Note dimple from pexing suture
Image courtesy of Shyamala Huilgol

Photo F Excellent outcome at 3 months with well-camouflaged scars and no eyelid oedema
Image courtesy of Shyamala Huilgol

QUESTION 4

Describe how you would perform a subcutaneous island pedicle flap for **Photo B,** including site-specific considerations.

Answer

1. Design: Draw along the nasolabial fold to the lower melolabial fold and from the lateral margin of the defect to meet at the lower melolabial fold, ensuring generous sizing (**Photo G**).

2. Administer an initial infra-orbital block and then cutaneous infiltration.

3. Using sterile technique, incise the flap to the deep subcutis. This depth is necessary to mobilise the flap on its pedicle but avoid incising the underlying muscle. Free the tail of the flap at the deep subcutis and undermine the leading edge of the flap in the superficial subcutis by 8–10 mm, leaving a central column of one-third or more of the flap length. Check the flap's movement. Consider deepening the inferior defect to permit the pedicle's entry and loosening the flap pedicle by cautious tunnelling at right angles to the flap with blunt-tipped scissors, being careful to avoid devitalising the flap. Undermine around the flap and defect in the mid-subcutaneous plane. Obtain haemostasis.

4. Insert a pexing suture 5–8 mm back from the undersurface of the flap's leading edge, to the infra-orbital periosteum to lift the flap into place and prevent ectropion. If the defect cannot be closed easily, close the

two leading corners of the flap in a "Pac-man" variant (**Photo H**) with cutaneous sutures only, increasing the effective length of the flap, then use an absorbable pexing suture to lift the flap into place. Consider partial closure of the primary defect with a dog ear (**Photo G**) to reduce its size. Use 5-0 buried absorbable sutures to close the inferior secondary defect (lift the lateral tissue slightly upwards to prevent puckering in the nasolabial fold), then the remainder of the flap. Place cutaneous sutures, ensuring good wound apposition (**Photo H**).

5. Give postoperative instructions, review for removal of sutures at one week and then longer term at 2–3 months. Encourage firm pressure application to the flap a few times daily with the tips of fingers or thumb from 2 weeks post-suture removal.

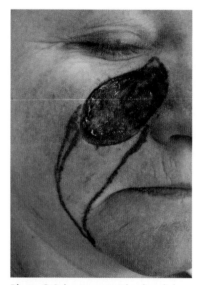 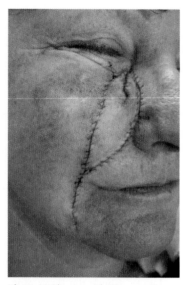

Photo G Subcutaneous island pedicle flap design with planned superior dog ear to reduce defect size. Line within the flap shows relaxed skin tension line.
Image courtesy of Shyamala Huilgol

Photo H Closure with "Pac-man" variation. The two "jaws" were not de-bevelled and were very lightly sutured with plans for later revision. Note indentation from pexing suture, below the "Pac-man" closure. A superior dog ear was removed below the eye.
Image courtesy of Shyamala Huilgol

QUESTION 5

What side effect has occurred in **Photo I,** and how would you manage this?

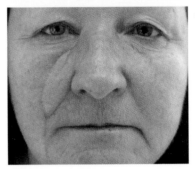

Photo I Subcutaneous island pedicle flap closure at 2 months
Image courtesy of Shyamala Huilgol

Answer

Pincushioning/trapdoor change

- Reassurance that this will improve.
- Encourage firm pressure application: 5–10 minutes, a few times daily, to swollen areas.
- Monthly triamcinolone acetonide injections (1 mL of 10 mg/mL) into the swollen areas (**Photo J**).
- Consider a series of three-monthly, fractionated ablative laser and subcision treatments (**Photos K** and **L**).

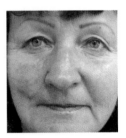

Photo J Result at 4 months after two triamcinolone injections
Image courtesy of Shyamala Huilgol

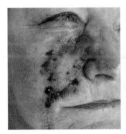

Photo K Immediately post fractionated ablative laser and subcision
Image courtesy of Shyamala Huilgol

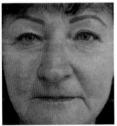

Photo L Excellent outcome at 4 months following laser and subcision revision, with resolution of scar indentation. Full face intense pulsed light (IPL) treatment was subsequently undertaken.
Image courtesy of Shyamala Huilgol

QUESTION 6

Describe how you would perform a Mustarde cheek rotation flap for **Photo C**, including site-specific considerations.

Answer

1. Design: draw laterally beneath the eye, then arc upwards and across the lateral canthus and temple, then follow the preauricular crease downwards. This increase in the radius of the flap lateral to the eye compensates for loss of flap height during rotation and acts to prevent downward secondary movement of the lower eyelid with ectropion. Place the dog ear along the nasolabial fold. Consider the need for a Burow's triangle below the ear (**Photo M**).

2. Consider perioperative antibiotics due to the flap size and extended operative time. Assess other risk factors for infection.

3. Perform infra-orbital and zygomaticofacial nerve blocks, then infiltrate locally. Consider as an alternative tumescent anaesthesia to both reduce pain and risk of local anaesthetic toxicity.

4. Using sterile technique, incise the flap and the medial aspect of the planned dog ear. Undermine in the mid-subcutaneous plane, including the flap and primary defect. One or two larger (cat's paw) skin hooks are helpful. Excise and undermine the Burow's triangle below the ear as needed. Obtain haemostasis. Place a 4-0 absorbable pexing suture from the deep edge of the flap and 6–10 mm behind its leading upper edge to the infra-orbital maxilla. Suspend the flap also at the temple with one or two 5-0 buried sutures so the flap is draped beneath the lower eyelid. Using 5-0 buried absorbable sutures, close the primary defect, with a horizontal tension vector to avoid ectropion. Remove the medial dog ear, then suture the flap into place with buried absorbable sutures. Consider leaving a 5 mm unsutured area in the lower pre-auricular or infra-auricular area or placing a drain to avoid a postoperative haematoma. Place cutaneous sutures with good wound apposition.

5. Give postoperative instructions, review for removal of sutures at one week (**Photo N**) and at 2–3 months (**Photos O** and **P**). Encourage firm pressure application to the flap a few times daily with the tips of fingers or thumb from approximately 2 weeks post-suture removal.

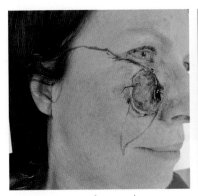

Photo M Design of Mustarde rotation flap with dog ear placed in the nasolabial fold
Image courtesy of Shyamala Huilgol

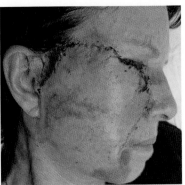

Photo N Mustarde flap at suture removal with acceptable anterior displacement of sideburn, desirable excess tissue beneath eyelid with good eyelid position. Note healing Burow's graft in upper pre-auricular, secondary defect
Image courtesy of Shyamala Huilgol

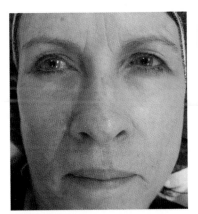

Photo O Excellent outcome at 3 months with good eyelid position and scar placement
Image courtesy of Shyamala Huilgol

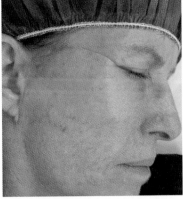

Photo P Lateral view at 3 months. Note displaced sideburn has been shaved. IPL was subsequently done for facial telangiectasia
Image courtesy of Shyamala Huilgol

Case 17
Duncan Stanford

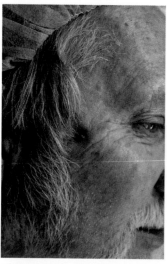

A 62-year-old man presents with a bleeding right zygoma lesion, treated with cryotherapy one year ago (**Photo A**).

Photo A Right zygoma lesion
Image courtesy of Duncan Stanford

QUESTION 1
What clinical findings would you assess?

Answer

- Size: 12 mm diameter
- Margins—poorly defined, no enhancement nor pearliness when stretched
- Palpation—indurated but not fixed to underlying tissue, including bone
- Cervical lymph nodes—not palpable (it could be an SCC)
- Full skin examination—other skin cancers are possible

QUESTION 2

How would you manage this lesion?

Answer

A biopsy (e.g. 4 mm punch) is needed for diagnosis and to assess high-risk features.

Comment

A shave or smaller punch biopsy may not give depth and growth pattern.

QUESTION 3

The biopsy report showed infiltrating BCC of 3.2 mm depth, into the deep subcutis. Is this a low- or high-risk BCC? List the factors you assessed.

Answer

High-risk BCC features are clinical (facial site, size >10 mm and poorly defined margins) and histological (infiltrating growth pattern and invasion below superficial subcutis).

QUESTION 4

What treatment options will you discuss with the patient? Discuss their pros and cons.

Answer

1. Mohs micrographic surgery. Its twin advantages are the high cure rate in combination with tissue conservation.

   The cure rate is greater than 98% at 5 years for primary BCC. The potential problem of incomplete excision when carrying out standard excision is avoided.

   The preservation of normal tissue assists with cosmesis, function (including avoidance of temporalis nerve damage) and simplifying reconstruction.

   Trained medical and lab personnel and a lab facility are required, hence, it's not always locally available. It may be too costly for some patients (most treatments are in the private day surgery or clinic setting) and the duration may make it impractical in elderly or frail patients.

2. Surgical excision with a wide excision margin. Surgical excision is the usual treatment for BCC and is widely available with many types of medical practitioners able to perform this procedure in a variety of healthcare settings, from general practitioner clinics to large teaching hospitals. Surgical margins are increased for higher risk tumours: in this case, 5 mm clinical margins will give a low incomplete excision rate at the lateral margins; increasing to 10 mm will further reduce this but require a more complex repair.

Audits suggest an incomplete excision rate of 10–15% following standard excision of facial tumours. Incomplete excision at the depth may be more likely in this case, attempting to avoid temporalis nerve damage.

If re-excision is required for positive margins, it may be difficult to determine which margin to re-excise, with potential for re-excision of the wrong margins or cosmetic and functional impairment if generous margins are taken. Higher risk tumours have higher recurrence rates, even with apparently complete excision. This is due to the sampling error inherent in standard processing with potential for missed positive margins. If recurrence is at the deep margin, delay in detection with an increased tumour size is common.

3. Radiotherapy. Radiotherapy has a good cure rate and is indicated in those keen to avoid surgery (including concerns about possible temporalis nerve damage) or when surgery is difficult (i.e. frail, elderly, anticoagulants, unstable heart disease with defibrillator, etc.).

Due to the usual late cosmetic outcomes (atrophy, telangiectasia, pigmentary change), it is not generally recommended below the age of 65. With hyperfractionation, the late radiodermatitis effects are reduced but the usual protocol (5 days per week for 4–6 weeks) is onerous, especially for rural or working patients. In frail individuals or where late cosmetic outcomes are immaterial, treatment can be given in a few fractions. There is always permanent local alopecia (important in the scalp and eyebrow). There will be inflammation and crusting during and after the treatment, though it is generally easy to manage and resolves after some weeks.

Radiotherapy requires expensive equipment and trained personnel and is thus only available in select locations. It is the least cost-effective method; however, free public hospital treatment and Medicare rebates in private settings mean that out-of-pocket costs may be similar to surgery.

Comment on alternatives

Other methods (e.g. cryotherapy, serial curettage and electrosurgery, photodynamic therapy, topical and injectable chemotherapy and immunostimulants) have an unacceptably low cure rate in this higher risk tumour and are contraindicated.

QUESTION 5

The tumour was cleared following two stages of Mohs surgery frozen sections stages and the defect measured 24× 26 mm (**Photo B**). What are your three preferred repair options?

Answer

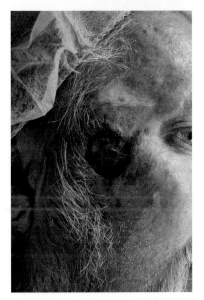

1. Side-to-side (curvilinear) closure—likely possible due to cheek/temple laxity (**Photo C**). Partial closure with a central Burow's full-thickness skin graft is a good "Plan B" if there is too much tension. The anterior Burow's triangle is both colour-matching and hairless, providing the better donor site of the two.

2. An advancement flap using preauricular laxity with lateral canthus dog ear removal is a standard and very good option.

Photo B Post-Mohs surgery defect
Image courtesy of Duncan Stanford

3. A transposition flap with recruitment of skin from the upper cheek and lateral lower eyelid with the dog ear removed inferolaterally. "Pointing" the flap at the eyelid will prevent ectropion, keeping movement parallel to the margin, and place the scar in natural lines.

Comment

Avoid crossing relaxed skin tension lines, moving hair-bearing skin into the defect or transecting the temporalis nerve.

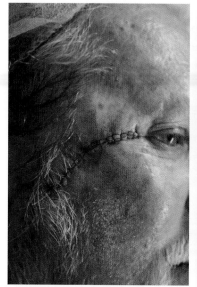

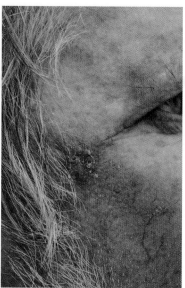

Photo C Shows result post-closure
Image courtesy of Duncan Stanford

Photo D Outcome at 6 weeks
Image courtesy of Duncan Stanford

Comment on alternatives

A rotation flap would effectively recruit lateral and lower cheek laxity but the dog ear would be placed in a less attractive inferior/anterior position. Transposition flaps using preauricular laxity would bring beard hair into the hairless zygoma region. An island pedicle flap from the inferior lateral cheek requires deep incisions and is relatively contraindicated due to potential for transection of the temporalis nerve and use of hair-bearing skin. A full-thickness graft will likely give a poor colour and contour match.

QUESTION 6

What complication is apparent in **Photo D** at the 6 week follow-up and what is the differential diagnosis?

Answer

Absorbable suture reaction (typical crusted papules). Other possibilities include infection, recurrence (too soon for a BCC) and new skin cancer.

Case 18
Simon Lee

An 84-year-old man underwent Mohs surgery for a primary infiltrative BCC involving the right central cheek. The final defect was 28 × 52 mm (**Photo A**).

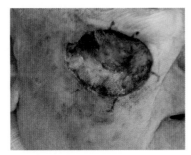

Photo A Post-Mohs surgery defect
Image courtesy of Simon Lee

QUESTION 1

What are your three favoured repair options? Comment on their relative merits.

Answer

1. Island pedicle flap
2. Rotation flap
3. Transposition flap

Comment

The lax skin is in the lower cheek and preauricular region.

- A large rotation or Mustarde flap would recruit skin from this area, while ensuring the direction of tension was horizontal and minimising downward tension on the eyelid. One or two pexing sutures would be required. A Burow's triangle below the ear would likely be needed to enhance flap movement. The defect would be closed across its long axis, generally a less preferred option. This is a larger procedure to perform under local anaesthesia, with significant postoperative bruising and swelling, particularly in the elderly. Tumescent anaesthesia may be very useful for these larger cases to reduce total dose and discomfort. In the late postoperative period, the flap often requires some corticosteroid injections to settle lower eyelid swelling above and bulkiness below the horizontal portion of the flap scar. Particular care must be taken with adequate sizing of the dog ear and sutured eversion of its edges to prevent obvious tissue redundancies and scar inversion in this more sebaceous cheek skin.

- This laxity may also be recruited with a transposition flap from the preauricular region with the pedicle in the superior position and the dog ear pointing towards the right temple. The vertical direction of flap closure tension would need careful management and pexing sutures to try and prevent ectropion, but this remains a risk. Transposition flaps often develop a degree of trapdooring. The usual steps should be taken to reduce this problem: correct flap sizing (do not undersize below the eye), undermining the defect edges, thinning the flap or increasing the defect's depth, pexing the flap to the base of the defect and using both deep and cutaneous sutures to ensure the flap edges are pulled down into the defect and everted. (A more favourable inferiorly based flap design is not possible in this case.) Post suture removal, the patient may apply firm pressure with the fingertips a few times daily to hasten the resolution of swelling. Triamcinolone acetonide (0.5–1.0 mL of 10 mg/mL) injections may be used as needed, monthly, from 6–8 weeks postoperatively. A series of three subcision and fractionated ablative laser treatments performed monthly are also very effective for indented cheek scarring (**Photos B and C**).

- An inferior and lateral subcutaneous island pedicle flap would involve the least amount of tissue movement and further tissue loss while closing the defect over the shortest aspect. However, this repair is the one most at risk of causing ectropion. At times, there is not as much subcutaneous tissue as anticipated and flap mobilisation can prove to be unexpectedly difficult. Trapdooring or pincushioning is also common with these flaps; preventive and treatment measures are discussed above.

Comment on alternatives

Primary closure is not possible. A full- or split-thickness graft will give a poor cosmetic outcome.

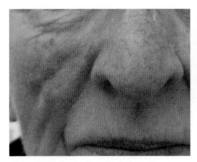

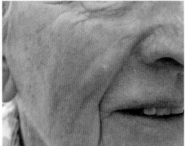

Photo B Indented and puckered cheek scar in sloping, horizontal limb of unilateral advancement flap. More vertical portion of scar lying in nasolabial fold is excellent.

Image courtesy of Shyamala Huilgol

Photo C Excellent outcome at 3 months following a series of three combined subcision and fractionated ablative laser treatments

Image courtesy of Shyamala Huilgol

QUESTION 2

A subcutaneous island flap with small Burow's graft repair is performed **(Photo D)**. What are your concerns regarding this repair?

Answer

There is some pull on the lower eyelid, but it is an oblique direction and is not causing significant displacement of the eyelid away from the globe.

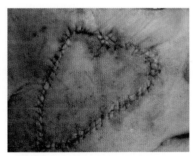

Photo D Subcutaneous island pedicle flap and small Burow's graft repair

Image courtesy of Simon Lee

QUESTION 3

What easy manoeuvre could you to do to assess this risk while performing the repair?

Answer

Once the flap is anchored in position with pexing and deep sutures, and before placing further sutures, the eyelid position is assessed under tension. The patient is requested to sit upright and look upwards while opening their mouth as wide as possible. If the lid margin remains apposed to the globe, then ectropion is less likely to develop. However, even when the flap has been adequately anchored to the orbital rim, unpredictable late contraction may still result in ectropion. The elderly often have preexisting eyelid laxity and are more vulnerable to this complication. Any patient having surgery near the eye must be consented for the possibility of ectropion.

QUESTION 4

What are the implications of not addressing this complication?

Answer

Ectropion often disrupts apposition of the lacrimal punctum to the globe, resulting in epiphora or excessive tears. In addition, the exposed conjunctiva may become dry and irritated, resulting in conjunctival inflammation. Very rarely, exposure keratopathy and impaired vision may occur.

QUESTION 5

The area heals well, but 2 months later the patient presents complaining of a "pore" at the lower medial suture margin that discharges a clear fluid, especially when eating. What is this complication and how should it be managed?

Answer

A parotid fistula is likely. Salivary discharge is typically stimulated by chewing or food smells. Many fistulae resolve spontaneously and initial conservative management with antibiotics, pressure dressings and serial aspiration is recommended. Anticholinergics and botulinum toxin injections may also be used to reduce salivary secretion and permit healing. Persistent fistulae require referral to a head and neck surgeon for identification (probing) and removal of the tract under anaesthesia.

Case 19
Gilberto Moreno Bonilla

A 65-year-old man with an indurated, biopsy-proven nodular BCC on the preauricular cheek has recently undergone successful spinal cord stimulator implantation for chronic lower back pain.

QUESTION 1

Discuss spinal cord stimulators, avoidance of electromagnetic interference with electrosurgical devices and potential complications from their use.

Answer

Spinal cord stimulators are implantable electronic devices (**Photo A**) and are sensitive to electromagnetic interference. Multiple brands exist with individualised recommendations, with no consensus perioperative guidelines available[1].

At initial consultation, ascertain the name, date and location of implant and its leads. Liaise with the managing specialist for perioperative management. Contact the industry representative and obtain the manufacturer's device brochure. It is safest to disable it for the surgery but ensure that symptoms will be tolerable. There may be on/off or surgery mode settings, under patient or physician control, possibly via an app. Patient consultation with the managing physician prior to and after surgery is advisable with postoperative evaluation and device interrogation by qualified personnel.

Avoid direct damage to the device and its leads and also overstretching of leads during patient positioning. Heat electrocautery (e.g. disposable Bovie high temperature cautery pen) generates no electrical current, avoids electrical interference and is the safest form of haemostasis. Bipolar (forceps) electrosurgery passes electrical current between the two tips, minimising electrical interference and potential damage to implanted electronic devices.

Electromagnetic interference from electrosurgery devices, specifically monopolar with grounding plate (e.g. Surgistat® with pointed tip) and monoterminal without grounding plate (e.g. older Hyfrecator® models), may cause harm to the patient (including death), damage the neurostimulator system or alter the programming. Current flow through the leads and electrode sites may result in permanent neural thermal injury, lead dislodgement, lead migration and tissue trauma, electrical shock, lead failure and device damage.

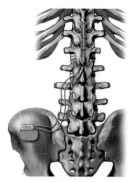

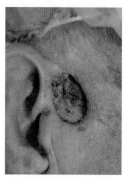

Photo A Implanted spinal neurostimulator
Source: Nucleus Medical Media Inc / Alamy Stock Photo

Photo B Post-Mohs surgery preauricular defect
Image courtesy of Gilberto Moreno Bonilla

QUESTION 2

Having followed appropriate precautions, the patient underwent Mohs surgery, resulting in a 26 × 18 mm defect **(Photo B)**. List three repair options and discuss their relative merits.

Answer

1. Advancement flap — Burow's triangle exchange or unilateral advancement (O–L) flap
2. Partial primary closure and Burow's graft
3. Rhombic transposition flap

Comment

• A Burow's triangle exchange flap is preferred. This robust flap moves the usual laxity from the lower cheek and jowls straight upwards. The vertical limb of the scar is hidden in the preauricular fold with the anterior Burow's triangle hidden in the hairline of the sideburn. The posterior Burow's triangle is placed unobtrusively below the earlobe but may be displaced to the point of extinction with the "rule of halves" to even the unequal sides in an O–L flap (**Photo C**).

- Partial primary closure of the lower defect may be combined with a Burow's graft to the upper defect in a simple repair. The graft will be slower to heal than a flap closure.

- A rhombic transposition flap recruits central cheek laxity, changing the direction of closure tension and creating a complex geometrical scar away from the favourable preauricular crease. The design and execution are more challenging, with potential for trapdooring and unanticipated secondary movement affecting the sideburn and beard.

Comment on alternatives

An island pedicle flap from below is possible but there is limited subcutaneous tissue and it may move less than anticipated. Care must also be taken in this area with deep motor nerves. A graft is a poorer option with likely suboptimal colour and texture match. Second intention healing is possible but will be slow and has some potential for chondritis of the nearby helical crus.

QUESTION 3

Outline execution of the Burow's triangle exchange advancement flap, following design, consent, local anaesthetic infiltration and sterile technique.

Answer

1. Incise the superior aspect of the upper Burow's triangle, preauricular crease and inferior aspect of the lower Burow's triangle (**Photo C**).

2. Undermine the flap, primary and secondary defects in the mid-subcutaneous plane, above the superficial musculoaponeurotic system (SMAS).

3. Confirm that the primary defect will close easily by lifting the flap with a skin hook, then excise both Burow's triangles.

4. Achieve haemostasis.

5. Close the primary defect first with a 5-0 buried absorbable suture to lift the flap superiorly (key suture), then close the lower Burow's triangle (secondary defect) and then the remainder of the flap with buried sutures.

6. Place 5-0 or 6-0 nylon cutaneous sutures (**Photo D**).

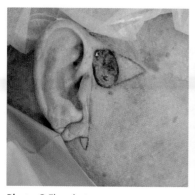 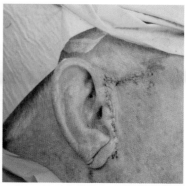

Photo C Flap design
Image courtesy of Gilberto Moreno Bonilla

Photo D Flap closure
Image courtesy of Gilberto Moreno Bonilla

QUESTION 4

What anatomic structures are at risk with this flap?

Answer

- Facial nerve branches (temporal and zygomatic), sitting below the SMAS but most superficial and vulnerable over the zygoma.
- Stensen's duct runs from the anterior parotid border, traverses the buccal fat pad, dives downwards at the anterior masseter border to enter the buccal mucosa at the second upper molar.
- Superficial parotid lobe lies beneath subcutaneous fat, over the masseter muscle, extending from the auditory meatus to the angle of the jaw and upper anterior neck.
- Superficial temporal artery and vein follow a tortuous course in the subcutaneous tissue, above the SMAS (both exposed in **Photo B**).
- Auriculotemporal nerve (one of three cutaneous branches of the mandibular nerve) emerges from the parotid and joins the superficial temporal vessels in the subcutaneous tissue.

Reference

1. Ghaly RF, Tverdohleb T, Candido KD, Knezevic NN. Do we need to establish guidelines for patients with neuromodulation implantable devices, including spinal cord stimulators undergoing nonspinal surgeries? Surg Neurol Int 2016 Feb 15; 7: 18.

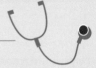

Section 5

Ears

Case 20
Nick Stewart

An 89-year-old woman underwent Mohs surgery for a biopsy-proven noduloinfiltrative BCC (**Photos A** and **B**) at the junction of the upper and middle thirds of the left helix, resulting in a 8 × 16 mm tumour-free defect (**Photo C**).

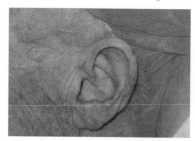

Photo A Anterior view of helical BCC
Image courtesy of Nick Stewart

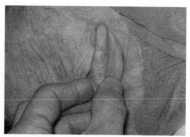

Photo B Superior view of helical BCC
Image courtesy of Nick Stewart

QUESTION 1
List three closure options for this defect in order of preference.

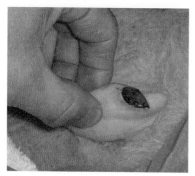

Photo C Superior view of helical defect
Image courtesy of Nick Stewart

Answer
1. Wedge repair
2. Full-thickness skin graft
3. Jelly roll flap[1]
4. Primary closure
5. Superior helical rim advancement flap — cutaneous or chondrocutaneous (Antia-Buch) variations with back-cut in upper rim and preauricular area.

6. Rotation flap along helical rim with back-cut in superior postauricular fold +/– conversion to double rotation flap
7. Bilobed flap

Comment

There are many options. Wedge excision is a standard repair for helical defects but will make the ear smaller. A full-thickness graft is often excellent when the underlying cartilage is intact but will be slower to heal than a flap. The jelly roll flap requires significant undermining but is otherwise a simple procedure and avoids thinning of the helical rim. The advancement, chondrocutaneous, rotation and bilobed flaps are possibly more complex than is needed for this smaller cutaneous defect. Chondrocutaneous flaps risk perichondrial haematoma (cauliflower ear). Primary closure will thin the helical rim, but this may be acceptable, especially in the elderly.

Comment on alternatives

An inferior helical rim advancement flap with its long pedicle risks necrosis. It is too far from the postauricular sulcus for a banner transposition flap. A two-stage interpolation flap is overly complex for this defect.

QUESTION 2

You elect to perform a stellate or staghorn wedge repair. Describe its design and advantage compared to a standard wedge repair.

Answer

A standard wedge repair is angled to a single apex of approximately 30° while the stellate variant has two additional 30° Burow's triangles, above and below (**Photo D**). This permits a larger defect to be closed with a reduced risk of anatomical distortion, particularly anterior or posterior buckling of the helix. Symmetry, both in the length of all sides and in the incisions through all layers of the helix, is paramount when planning and executing both the standard wedge and the stellate variant.

QUESTION 3
What are the key sutures for this repair?

Answer

The cartilage is closed first, starting with the three triangles and finishing with the helical rim, using either 5-0 absorbable (e.g. Monosyn™) or colourless non-absorbable (e.g. Prolene™) buried sutures. The latter has the dual advantage of low-tissue reactivity and maintaining long-term tensile strength, reducing the risk of late-onset cartilage separation. The knots are positioned on the posterior aspect of the cartilage, where they are less likely to cause discomfort. The anterior and posterior cutaneous aspects are closed with 5-0 or 6-0 nylon sutures, using everting sutures (e.g. vertical or horizontal mattress sutures) and/or Z-plasties at the helical rim to minimise the risk of helical rim notching (**Photo E**).

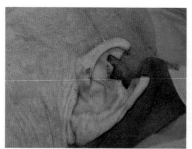 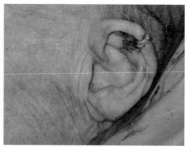

Photo D Stellate wedge repair prior to closure
Image courtesy of Nick Stewart

Photo E Stellate repair post closure. Note everting mattress sutures at the helical rim.
Image courtesy of Nick Stewart

QUESTION 4

The patient presents for follow-up after 10 weeks and complains of a painful nodule near the area of the surgery. List four potential causes of a postoperative nodule on the ear.

Answer

1. Chondrodermatitis nodularis helicis
2. Suture granuloma
3. Hypertrophic/keloid scarring
4. Perichondrial haematoma

Comment on alternatives

Tumour recurrence from BCC is highly unlikely at such an early date and is unlikely to present with pain. It is common for patients to notice some ear tenderness for 2–3 months after ear surgery but this does not present with a nodule and usually settles spontaneously. Surgeons should ensure they provide preoperative and postoperative education and ask patients to return if the problem does not resolve.

QUESTION 5

You suspect chondrodermatitis nodularis helicis (CNH). What is the aetiology of this condition?

Answer

CNH is a painful, inflammatory reaction caused by repeated pressure on the skin and underlying cartilage, most commonly during sleep. Other contributing factors include poor blood supply, cold, sun exposure, trauma and connective tissue diseases.

Following surgery, it is most likely due to insufficient or uneven removal of cartilage with protuberant areas being prone to developing this problem. As a spontaneous problem, it most commonly occurs as a result of sleeping on the affected side, but is also caused by pressure from hearing aids, headphones, CPAP mask straps, wimples, etc. When caused by sleeping, it occurs on the most protuberant aspect of the helix or antihelix, and the patient is often woken during the night with an aching pain. The patient usually preferentially sleeps on the affected side due to habitual or biomechanical reasons (e.g. contralateral hip or shoulder problems).

QUESTION 6

How do you manage this complication?

Answer

When CNH arises after surgery, simple measures may be tried first but surgical revision is likely to be needed. In idiopathic situations, an explanation of the aetiology, along with simple measures to remove pressure (e.g. avoiding sleeping on the affected side, using a donut pillow or foam inserts into pillow cases, adherent bunion pads at night) may be adequate. Topical corticosteroids (e.g. 0.05% betamethasone dipropionate ointment) or intralesional steroids (e.g. triamcinolone acetonide 10 mg/mL) offer quicker relief and may be used in combination with previous measures to remove pressure.

Surgical revision is usually reserved for cases refractory to the above treatments, or when there is obvious distortion of the underlying cartilage, such as may arise post surgical excision. In addition to the standard risks of cutaneous surgery, surgical revision has the added disadvantage of potentially shifting the problem to the next most protuberant area, so particular care must be taken to ensure a smooth contour in the underlying cartilage. Postoperatively, removable pressure issues should again be addressed.

Topical 2% nitroglycerin paste, hyaluronic fillers, diltiazem cream and liquid nitrogen cryotherapy have also been described as treatment measures.

Reference
1. Wentzell JM, Wisco OJ. The helix jelly roll flap. Dermatol Surg 2010; 36: 1183–1190.

Case 21
Richard Turner

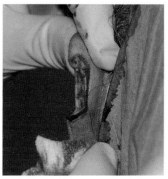

A 71-year-old man with a well-defined BCC on the helical rim was managed by standard excision with 4 mm margins, including helical cartilage to ensure clearance at the depth. The defect measured 7 × 12 mm (**Photo A**).

Photo A Defect following tumour excision

Image courtesy of Richard Turner

QUESTION 1

List the repair options for this defect. Outline their relative advantages and disadvantages.

Answer

1. Wedge excision
2. Helical rim advancement flap
3. Two-stage interpolation flap

Wedge excision is a reliable closure with good results for smaller rim defects. It reduces the size of the ear and may cause some anterior cupping of the ear; both are more likely with larger excisions. The incision into the conchal bowl changes its shape, possibly interfering with hearing aids and glasses. Potential longer-term issues include rim notching and antihelix irregularity with a risk of chondrodermatitis. Two-stage interpolated flaps raising retroauricular skin in conjunction with cartilage strutting are helpful, especially with larger full-thickness rim defects, but require multiple attendances. This complex repair is not warranted for this smaller defect. The helical rim advancement flap reliably re-creates the curved rim shape, while avoiding changes to the conchal bowl and distortion of the overall ear shape, and is the preferred reconstruction.

Comment on alternatives

Second intention healing and skin grafting will give a poor cosmetic outcome with a large visible notch. Side-to-side closure along the curvature of the ear will remove the helical rim but the smaller width and flatter ear may be acceptable in selected patients.

QUESTION 2

Describe the differences between classical and modified helical rim advancement flap designs, including their relative merits.

Answer

The classical approach (full thickness) detaches the entire helical rim anteriorly and posteriorly to directly close the defect. This quick and easy repair takes advantage of the reliable blood supply to the rim from the superior and inferior auricular arteries. The flap is narrow with a greater risk of tip necrosis and subsequent notching, especially if there is excessive tension or if the incision extends into the inferior auricular artery. Commonly, there is some thinning of the helical rim at the closure site.

In the modified approach (partial thickness), only the anterior skin and cartilage are incised in the helical rim sulcus, leaving posterior helical skin intact; undermining of the posterior pinna is followed by advancement and closure. The broader-based and larger flap is very reliable, but requires more skill to execute and has a greater risk of haematoma and wound infection. The standing cone on the posterior ear needs to be excised, thus the flap can be particularly useful if the defect extends posteriorly. Cupping of the ear may occur, especially with larger defects.

Both techniques use a Burow's triangle in the anterior earlobe to increase flap movement with a resultant reduction in lobe size and ear height.

A second, superiorly based back-cut chondrocutaneous flap may be added to an inferior modified helical advancement flap in the Antia-Buch repair.

QUESTION 3
Describe how you would perform the repair.

Answer

1. After marking the repair and obtaining informed consent, anaesthetise the ear from the postauricular sulcus to the rim, including the lobe.
2. Using sterile technique, incise in the sulcus between helix and antihelix, from the lower anterior defect to the lobe. Cut through any underlying cartilage in the helical sulcus but leave the posterior ear skin intact. Remove a Burow's triangle in the anterior earlobe to increase flap mobility and reach (**Photo B**).
3. Undermine carefully between the cartilage and posterior ear skin, extending to the postauricular sulcus, then undermine the lobe, splitting it in the subcutaneous plane (**Photo C**).
4. Achieve haemostasis, then advance the flap and close the defect. Use a 5-0 absorbable vertical mattress suture to oppose the inferior flap to the superior defect margin and carefully re-create the fossa between the helix and antihelix. If the flap is under tension, consider excising a thin crescent of cartilage on the outside edge of the ear to reduce the distance the flap must stretch. Use further buried vertical mattress sutures to close the primary and secondary defects, including the Burow's triangle.
6. Excise the standing cone on the posterior pinna. Take care not to remove too much tissue over the convexity of the posterior ear to avoid buckling.
7. To avoid notching of the rim, insert 2 or 3 cutaneous vertical mattress sutures to create exaggerated eversion of the helical rim. Close the remaining defect with running cutaneous sutures, 5-0 nylon or polypropylene (**Photo D**).
8. Apply petrolatum jelly and a simple non-stick dressing. The patient should be provided with contact details, written instructions and adequate analgesics. Postoperative ice packs reduce pain, swelling and the risk of postoperative bleeding. Pressure to the back of the ear may be provided by padding, removed after 48 hours. Infection, particularly *Pseudomonas*, is more common on the ear and prophylactic antibiotics

(ciprofloxacin or cephalexin) should be considered if risk factors are present. Finally, the patient should be warned that the visible eversion of the wound edges at the rim should settle after suture removal.

9. Remove sutures at 7–10 days and review again at 3 months (**Photo E**).

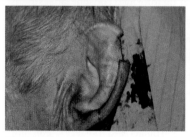

Photo B Flap incision along the helical sulcus with a Burow's triangle in the lobe
Image courtesy of Richard Turner

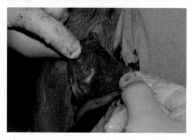

Photo C Extensive undermining of posterior ear
Image courtesy of Richard Turner

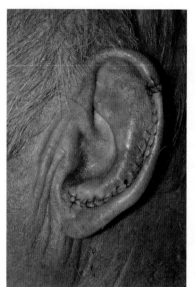

Photo D Completed repair
Image courtesy of Richard Turner

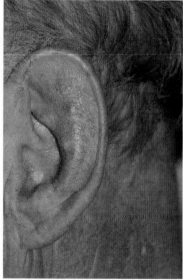

Photo E Excellent result at 3 months
Image courtesy of Richard Turner

Case 22
Shyamala Huilgol

A 79-year-old man underwent Mohs surgery for a poorly defined nodular BCC on the left ear conchal bowl. The resultant defect measured 15 × 15 mm and had excision of the underlying cartilage (**Photo A**).

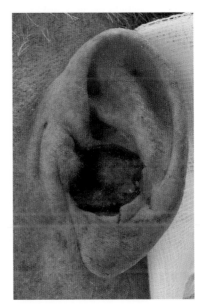

Photo A Postoperative conchal defect with excision of underlying cartilage
Image courtesy of Shyamala Huilgol

QUESTION 1
What are your three favoured repair options?

Answer
1. Pull through island flap
2. Full-thickness graft
3. Split-thickness graft

Comment on alternatives

Second intention healing is possible but will be prolonged and may cause stenosis of the external auditory canal with functional consequences and/ or cosmetic distortion of the external ear.

QUESTION 2

List split-thickness donor sites and discuss their relative merits.

Answer

Mastoid scalp, upper arm, anterior thigh.

The scalp is much quicker to heal than the alternatives (usually healed at 2 weeks), scars minimally and hair grows back quickly to cover the area. Hairy donor sites must be shaved, thus the scalp is usually unsuitable for those with long hair as regrowth and disfigurement will be prolonged. The arm and thigh are prone to prolonged healing, particularly in individuals with underlying health issues, and there will initially be a dark, red scar that then turns white, which may be very noticeable in tanned skin. Hypertrophic scarring may result, particularly on the upper arm. Dressing care is easiest on the thigh, but it seems most prone to significant postoperative pain.

QUESTION 3

Describe how you would plan and execute a pull through flap.

Answer

Design: Make a template of the defect with a suture packet or other sterile non-stretch material (**Photo B**). Check the template size again before proceeding to ensure the flap is neither under nor over sized. Use this template to design a donor site centred on the post-auricular sulcus (**Photo C**), lying immediately behind the defect. Remember to maintain the correct orientation for the template: the flap will be swung through the ear, thus the lateral posterior flap will end up on the medial anterior defect. Dog ears are drawn above and below the donor site, which is usually closed in a linear fashion.

Execution: Infiltrate local anaesthesia to both aspects of the ear. Using sterile technique, the flap is incised and peripherally undermined, leaving the central deep pedicle in the retroauricular sulcus intact (**Photo D**). If the cartilage is missing throughout the entire defect, as in this case, the hemicircle of the flap on the helical side is aligned with the defect's margins on the helical side and the flap is swung through like a revolving door (**Photos D and E**). In other cases, with only central loss of the cartilage, the flap is folded in half, pulled through a central incision and then unfolded. Following haemostasis, the flap is sutured anteriorly with 6-0 cutaneous sutures. The secondary defect is then closed, usually with excision of superior and inferior dog ears and a linear closure in the retroauricular sulcus. In this case, the defect was quite wide and so it was repaired with a combination of a transposition flap from the superior retroauricular sulcus and an advancement flap from the infra-auricular neck (**Photos F and G**). Excellent results were achieved at long-term follow-up (**Photo H**).

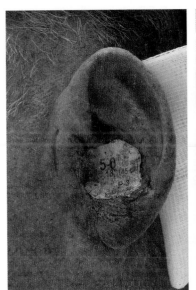

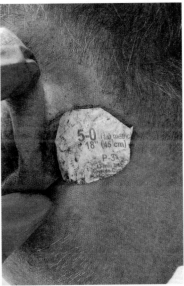

Photo B Template of defect made with suture packet

Image courtesy of Shyamala Huilgol

Photo C Template over flap site in retroauricular sulcus. Correct orientation of the template is essential.

Image courtesy of Shyamala Huilgol

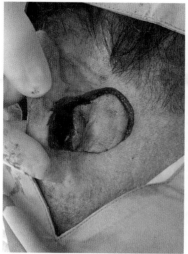

Photo D Flap incised. The helical border of both anterior defect and posterior flap are the same.

Image courtesy of Shyamala Huilgol

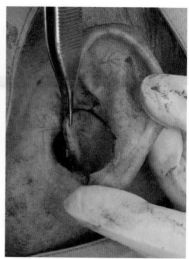

Photo E Flap being pulled through

Image courtesy of Shyamala Huilgol

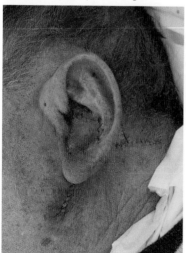

Photo F Flap sutured in place

Image courtesy of Shyamala Huilgol

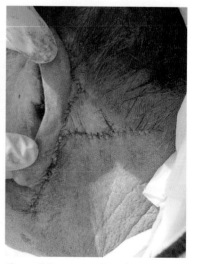

Photo G Rear view of combined transposition and advancement flap repairs of secondary defect

Image courtesy of Shyamala Huilgol

QUESTION 4

This man has atrial fibrillation and is taking oral apixaban for prevention of stroke and systemic embolism. Describe your perioperative management of all anticoagulants and supplements.

Answer

Complex surgery, particularly on the head and neck, generally requires perioperative management of anticoagulants, while simple non-facial closures usually do not. Consult with the prescribing doctor before stopping or altering anticoagulants in patients with existing medical conditions.

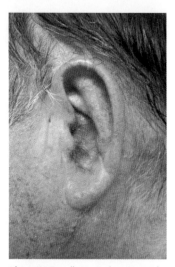

Photo H Excellent result at 3 months
Image courtesy of Shyamala Huilgol

- Aspirin: Continue for secondary prevention. Discontinue 10–14 days preop if no medical indication.
- Aspirin/clopidogrel combination: Stop clopidogrel and use aspirin only 7 days preop. Restart combined treatment 24–48 hours postop.
- Clopidogrel: Continue if single-agent use.
- Aspirin/ticagrelor combination: Cease ticagrelor 5 days preop, recommence 24 hours postop.
- Warfarin: Check INR within 4 days of surgery and aim to have ≤ 3. If > 3.5, stop for 2 days preop and recheck INR one day preop.
- Warfarin/aspirin combination: Liaise with treating physician – if possible, stop aspirin. If combined therapy must continue, reduce warfarin dose to have INR at 2–2.5.
- Apixaban: Cease 2 days preop, recommence 24 hours postop.
- Dabigatran or rivaroxaban: Cease 1 day preop, recommence 24 hours postop.
- Non-steroidal anti-inflammatory medications: Cease 3 days preop.
- Supplements (fish oil, garlic, ginkgo biloba, ginseng, ginger, vitamin E, feverfew): Cease one week preop.
- Alcohol: Cease 1–2 days preop, remain abstinent for 1–2 days postop.

Case 23
Duncan Stanford

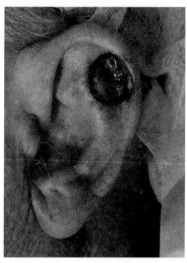

A 66-year-old man had a 15 × 19 mm left ear scaphoid fossa defect after clearance of an infiltrative BCC by Mohs micrographic technique **(Photo A)**.

Photo A Left ear scaphoid fossa defect
Image courtesy of Duncan Stanford

QUESTION 1
List four repair options you would discuss with this patient.

Answer
1. Full-thickness skin graft
2. Split-thickness skin graft
3. Second intention healing
4. Chondrocutaneous rotation flap

QUESTION 2

Briefly discuss the pros and cons for each repair option. Discuss donor site options for any grafts.

Answer

1. Full-thickness skin graft: preferred donor site — ipsilateral postauricular sulcus, unless a good reason to avoid this such as previous surgery or suspicious lesions. Good colour and contour match likely with the postauricular donor site, which is also easy to close, manage (as close to graft site) and heal.

   May have some graft pincushioning if the donor skin is thicker than the depth of the defect. Colour mismatch is uncommon with a postauricular donor but also unlikely to be of concern in this site. Graft failure is uncommon. Ipsilateral preauricular sulcus less favoured — poorer colour and thickness match. Need to take care to avoid transferring male beard hair to the ear.

2. Split-thickness skin graft: simple repair with excellent take rate, minimal contraction when cartilage is intact (as in this case) so cosmetic outcome likely to be good. A thigh or upper arm donor site is sometimes troublesome with pain and slow healing; in men and women with short hair, the author prefers the shaved postauricular scalp with its dual benefits of rapid healing and hidden scarring. Graft failure is uncommon (usually due to bleeding or infection) but partial failure with prolonged healing may occur.

3. Second intention: fenestration of the cartilage with 2 mm punch excisions would speed healing. A good cosmetic outcome is likely. The benefit is less surgery but at the cost of more prolonged wound care. *Pseudomonas* chondritis is always a risk when cartilage is left exposed for a prolonged period.

4. Cutaneous or chondrocutaneous rotation flap: given the defect size, a bilateral design will be needed and a standing cone may need to be excised from the earlobe. The chief benefit is more rapid healing than a graft or second intention; further, the size of the ear is not significantly reduced, unlike a wedge. The surgery is more complex than the alternatives, helical distortion is possible and any excision of cartilage usually results in tenderness for a few months. Chondrodermatitis nodularis is always

possible when there is excision of cartilage and potential for pressure on prominent areas along the reshaped antihelix.

Comment on alternatives

Wedge resection is less favoured as the ear rim and cartilage are intact. This repair will shrink the height of the ear, forward cupping of the smaller ear to at least a small extent is common and a few months of postoperative tenderness following any surgery to cartilage is usual. Chondrodermatitis nodularis helicis is again possible.

An interpolation flap from preauricular skin is unnecessarily complex with its need for two surgical procedures.

A pull-through island pedicle flap is not usually undertaken where perichondrium and cartilage are intact and this defect is too far from the postauricular sulcus for the standard flap design.

A transposition flap is not possible, as the defect is too far from the earlobe.

QUESTION 3

Describe the steps in performing a full-thickness graft repair, including design, technique, suture materials, dressings and follow-up.

Answer

1. Evaluate the defect: most of the cartilage is intact in this case but consider a few 2 mm punch excisions through the cartilage (to increase vascularisation and "take" rate).
2. Measure the defect and make a template using a non-stick dressing (e.g. Telfa®). Plan to oversize the graft by about 5–10% as it will shrink after harvesting.
3. Place the template on the donor area and draw an ellipse around it. Anaesthetise this area.
4. Some surgeons will perforate the graft while still *in situ* in the donor area using an 18 gauge needle (to reduce collection of fluid beneath the graft and hence improve the "take" rate).
5. Harvest the graft and place in sterile saline. Undermine the donor site edges then secure haemostasis. Some surgeons may place buried

sutures (e.g. 4-0 or 5-0 poliglecaprone 25 [Monocryl®] or polyglactin 910 [Vicryl]®), first while others place only a percutaneous running horizontal mattress suture with low tissue drag for easy removal (e.g. 4-0 or 5-0 polybutester or polypropylene) **(Photo B)**.

6. Remove the graft from the sterile saline and defat.

7. Ensure haemostasis at the recipient site, then suture the graft into place using a fine (5-0 or 6-0) non-absorbable interrupted (or running) nylon or polypropylene suture **(Photo C)**. Some surgeons would use an absorbable suture (e.g. glycolide-lactide [Vicryl Rapide®]) or glyconate (Monosyn Quick®), especially if the patient will have difficulty returning for suture removal. Use the "ship-to-shore" and "shallow bite, deep bite" technique to "recess" the graft into the bed. Ensure precise wound edge approximation.

8. A tie-over bolster dressing or pexing sutures can be used to ensure firm adhesion of the graft to the bed. For the bolster option, apply white soft petrolatum to the graft, then a non-stick dressing (e.g. petrolatum gauze or other non-adherent dressing) [Telfa®/Melolin®] and then the cotton wool bolster. The bolster is moulded to shape and tied over with four long sutures (e.g. 4-0 silk). Finally, cover with a firm pressure dressing. The bolster will be soaked with sterile saline for 10 minutes, prior to removal when the patient returns for suture removal in 7 days.

9. Alternatively, the dressing may be removed after 2 days followed by cautious daily cleansing, the reapplication of petrolatum and a non-stick dressing. Some practitioners simply leave the graft open at this stage and apply petrolatum twice daily.

10. Review for a wound check in 2 days (ideally) and removal of sutures in 7 days (unless absorbable suture used percutaneously). Delay suture removal if the graft is discoloured or has not fully taken. Review the outcome at about 6–10 weeks **(Photo D)** when cosmetic issues can be assessed and management options discussed. As always, ensure a total body skin check is organised for 4–6 months.

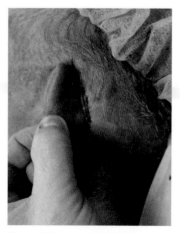

Photo B Postauricular donor site
Image courtesy of Duncan Stanford

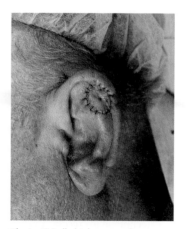

Photo C Full-thickness graft sewn in place with central pexing suture
Image courtesy of Duncan Stanford

QUESTION 4
List five risks or complications that you would discuss with this patient.

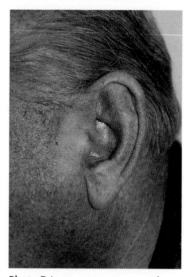

Photo D Long-term outcome with excellent colour and contour match. Note very minor internal helical rim distortion, due to focal helical tissue loss during tumour excision.
Image courtesy of Duncan Stanford

Answer
1. Graft failure: partial or full thickness. Most commonly due to bleeding or infection.
2. Bleeding: may result in haemorrhage or haematoma.
3. Infection: at graft or donor site.
4. Graft mismatch: in colour/texture/contour.
5. Helical rim notching: due to contraction (especially if graft failure).

Comment on alternatives
Seroma or collection is unlikely at this site.

Case 24
Duncan Stanford

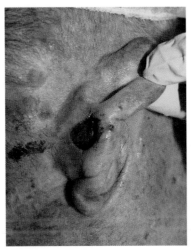

An 82-year-old man underwent Mohs surgery for an ill-defined recurrent nodular BCC on the posterior ear close to the mid-helix. The defect size following clearance of the tumour measured 12 × 12 mm **(Photo A)**.

Photo A Posterior ear defect close to mid-helix
Image courtesy of Duncan Stanford

QUESTION 1
List four repair options you would discuss with this patient and discuss their advantages and disadvantages.

Answer

1. Double rotation flap—A flap permits more rapid healing than a graft and a broad-based rotation flap has better perfusion than flaps with narrow pedicles. A double rotation or anchor flap design is preferable to a single rotation flap, the mid-ear defect position permitting recruitment of laxity from both upper and lower ear. Extension to

the postauricular sulcus permits recruitment of laxity from this area. (Opposing flap directions with an O–Z design is useful when the defect abuts the postauricular sulcus.)

Flaps on the posterior ear sometimes lead to permanent loss of sensation due to damage to the limited number of sensory nerve branches from the great auricular nerve. Care must be taken with haemostasis as damage to larger postauricular blood vessels during undermining may lead to bleeding and haematoma.

2. Banner or rhombic transposition flap from postauricular sulcus—A simple flap design recruiting from a predictable area of laxity in the postauricular sulcus. An inferior base is preferable to a superior base as it will be less likely to pincushion. Care must be taken to correctly size the flap as the donor area is commonly under tension and the flap will contract after it is cut; hence, the flap width may be less than anticipated. A banner flap length-to-width ratio should be no more than 3:1 to permit good perfusion while also permitting closure of the secondary defect. There will be some lessening of the depth of the postauricular sulcus; if marked, this may tether the ear to the scalp and may be problematic in patients with larger, old-fashioned hearing aids or with the retroauricular arm portion of certain eye glasses.

3. Second intention—A good cosmetic outcome is likely, and this is also an inconspicuous site. The benefit is less surgery but at the cost of more prolonged wound care. Pseudomonas chondritis is always a risk when cartilage is left exposed for a prolonged period. The risk of contraction distorting helical rim curvature is low as the cartilage is intact and the defect some distance from rim. Fenestration of the cartilage with 2 mm punch excisions would speed healing.

4. Full-thickness skin graft (postauricular donor)—A good uncomplicated repair with likely good "take" and cosmetic outcome given modest defect size and depth.

Comment on alternatives

Primary closure will buckle cartilage and probably dehisce. Partial closure combined with a Burow's graft is more useful for defects in or near the sulcus.

A split-thickness skin graft with a mastoid donor site is often a reasonable option but has greater donor site morbidity than a full-thickness graft and is not needed for this modest defect.

A bilobed transposition flap is not needed given the proximity of defect to sulcus but is helpful in defects placed further from the sulcus.

Wedge resection is not necessary as the helical cartilage is intact. This repair would reduce the vertical height of the ear with a tendency to forwards cupping of the ear. It also changes the shape of the ear with protuberant cartilage prone to later nodular chondro-dermatitis.

Advancement flaps (e.g. Burow's exchange or T-plasty) will produce less movement than a rotation design in this case.

Interpolation flaps are unnecessarily complex.

Island pedicle flaps will not easily move away from the postauricular sulcus and are therefore a better option when the defect abuts the postauricular sulcus. They are usually subcutaneous but may have a muscular pedicle component if there is a well-developed posterior auricularis muscle. An inferior design taps into considerable laxity behind the earlobe.

QUESTION 2

You elect to perform a double rotation flap. Describe the steps in performing this repair, including design, technique, suture materials, dressings and follow-up.

Answer

1. Given the more lateral location of the defect, the flap arcs run around the posterior edge of the rim both superiorly and inferiorly from the lateral defect margin. The flap may be designed with a standing cone or Burow's triangle based on the medial defect edge, extending towards the sulcus with an apical angle about 30 degrees. Alternatively, the standing cone may be removed only after the flap arms are apposed. This option may be better as the convexity of the posterior ear may lead to overestimation of the amount of skin that is surplus and that may be safely removed.

2. Incise the flap and undermine above the perichondrium, and then ensure complete haemostasis, paying particular care to larger postauricular blood vessels.

3. Close the primary defect with buried or cutaneous sutures to create two secondary crescentic defects, each of which is then closed using the "rule of halves" and spreading the tension over the entire flap. Minimising the use of 5-0 absorbable sutures (e.g. polyglecaprone or polyglyconate) will reduce the risk of a deep suture reaction in this thin skin. After

trimming redundant skin at the curved tips, a partially buried mattress suture through both flap tips can be placed. Interrupted or running cutaneous sutures (e.g. 5-0 or 6-0 nylon or polypropylene) are used to precisely approximate wound edges with good eversion (**Photo B**).

4. Apply petrolatum to the suture line and then a non-stick dressing (e.g. Telfa®). Apply pressure layers (e.g. folded gauze) and then an adherent layer (e.g. Hypafix®) to hold it in place.

5. Consider prophylactic antibiotics, such as cephalexin or ciprofloxacin (ideally started at least 1 hour preop), if there is immunosuppression or other predisposing factors to infection, given the ear site.

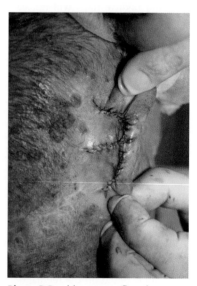

6. Discuss aftercare and provide printed instructions including restriction of activities, ice packs, analgesia and wound care along with contact details, including after-hours phone numbers.

7. Consider a wound check at 2 days to remove the pressure dressing and commence open care or patient-led dressings. Suture removal is at 7–10 days, with flap review at 6–12 weeks (**Photo C**). Ensure that a general skin check is organised.

Photo B Double rotation flap closure
Image courtesy of Duncan Stanford

QUESTION 3

List the side effects and complications you would discuss when gaining consent from the patient for any of your proposed repairs at the preoperative consultation.

Answer
1. Pain—local anaesthetic administration; postoperative including chondritis
2. Swelling
3. Bruising

4. Sensory change—flaps can be numb for weeks to months but rarely longer or permanently. Permanent numbness is more likely with undermining of postauricular skin and damage to branches of the great auricular nerve. Transient dysaesthesia is common during reinnervation

5. Bleeding

6. Haematoma/seroma

7. Infection

8. Dehiscence

9. Flap or graft necrosis

10. Poor cosmesis—rim notching and cupping (unlikely with correct design of this flap). Keloid or hypertrophic scarring may need treatment. Scarring and graft mismatch less conspicuous here

11. Functional impairment—difficulty wearing spectacles, hearing aids and face masks are all unlikely with the proposed repairs

12. Recurrence—this is unlikely after Mohs surgery with its 96% 5-year cure rate for recurrent BCC. Future treatment will be required if this occurs.

Comment

Incomplete excision requiring immediate further management is a significant risk when using standard excision margins and standard breadloaf pathology sectioning, especially with recurrent and poorly defined tumours on the ear.

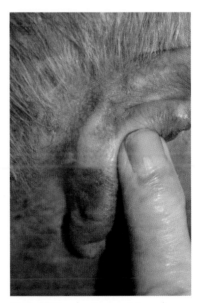

Photo C Good outcome at 6 weeks
Image courtesy of Duncan Stanford

Section 6
Periocular

Case 25
Paul Cherian and Shyamala Huilgol

A 76-year-old man with a nodular BCC on the right medial canthus and nasal root underwent Mohs surgical excision with a final defect of 15 × 21 mm (**Photos A** and **B**).

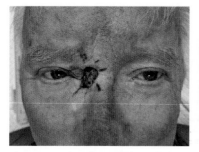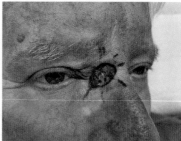

Photos A and **B** The medial canthus and nasal root defect
Image courtesy of Paul Cherian

QUESTION 1
What are your four favoured repair options? Comment on their relative merits.

Answer

1. Transposed island pedicle flap — Potential for bulkiness at pedicle rotation point.
2. Banner transposition flap — Potential for unanticipated secondary vectors of movement with consequent distortion.
3. Glabellar back-cut rotation flap (medially based) — Back-cut may be excised to prevent unattractive Y-shaped scar in the glabellar area, but increases the risk of bringing brows noticeably closer together. Webbing across the nasal root concavity is also a potential complication of this repair.

Comment

All three proposed flaps recruit matching skin from the adjacent glabellar cosmetic unit and permit the donor scar to be oriented within existing glabellar rhytids. The transposed island flap has a low risk of producing brow distortion, while the banner and back-cut rotation flaps have a greater risk for distortion and bringing brows too close together. The transposed island and transposition flaps have greater risks for pincushioning.

4. Full-thickness skin graft – A less technically challenging repair. Potential for poor skin match between the donor site and recipient site. Greater potential for partial failure compared to a flap with consequences of contracture, webbing and distortion of the medial canthus, eyelid and lacrimal structures.

Comment on alternatives

The defect is too large for second intention healing—webbing or tenting across the canthal and nasal root depressions is likely. It is too large to use a horizontal island pedicle flap across the nasal root. A classic rhombic flap would induce brow distortion. A bilobed flap from the glabella will leave the tertiary defect closure line at odds with natural glabellar creases. A transposition flap from the nasofacial sulcus will have a rotation pucker excision poorly located overlying the medial canthal tendon and lacrimal structures.

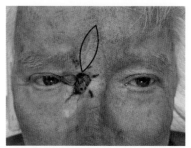

Photo C Design of flap. The width of the flap is equal to the vertical height of the defect.
Image courtesy of Paul Cherian

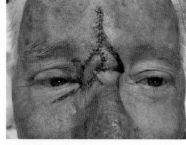

Photo D Post repair
Image courtesy of Paul Cherian

QUESTION 2

You decide to perform a transposed island pedicle flap (**Photos C** and **D**). Pincushioning and pedicle bulkiness are flap-specific potential problems. How can you minimise them?

Answer

Pincushioning of the flap can be reduced through slight undersizing of the flap, selective undermining of the recipient site (to allow even dispersion of scar tension), careful pexing of the flap to the underlying nasalis muscle with absorbable sutures and differential thinning of the flap.

Care must be taken not to compromise the vascular supply of the flap. Check for blanching of the flap when inserting the pexing suture. If the flap blanches, release the pexing suture and attempt a more superficial reinsertion.

The transposed pedicle flap is bulky in its medial-most portion by necessity (as it contains the nutrient pedicle). Fortunately, in this case, the glabellar aspect of the defect is deeper than the canthal aspect of the defect. The flap was thinned differentially to approximate the different depths of the defect. The early and final outcomes were excellent (**Photos E** and **F**).

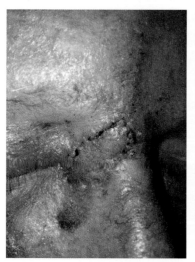 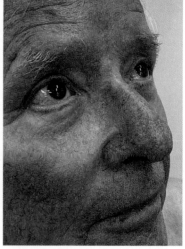

Photo E Early result at one week
Image courtesy of Paul Cherian

Photo F Result at 6 months. Note excellent matching to surrounding skin and absence of any distortion.
Image courtesy of Paul Cherian

QUESTION 3

The patient complained of troublesome epiphora at suture removal (**Photo E**). How would you manage this?

Answer

Early postoperative epiphora in this site is quite common and most often due to postoperative swelling, with pressure on the lacrimal ducts creating a temporary partial blockage. It is possible also that swelling is lifting the tear duct puncta away from the globe—examine and document this if present. Given the relatively mild swelling in this case, the latter issue is less likely.

Explanation to the patient of the likely temporary nature of this problem is essential along with reassurance that you will review the issue at 3 months. If it persists, it is worth injecting a small amount of intralesional triamcinolone on two occasions, a month apart. Persistence beyond this should prompt referral to an oculoplastic surgeon. Syringing of the duct may be all that is required but lacrimal duct surgery may also be needed. Lacrimal duct blockages are common in the elderly population. It is therefore helpful to ask about and document this issue preoperatively when operating near the eye as part of obtaining informed consent.

Case 26
Duncan Stanford, Dinesh Selva and Shyamala Huilgol

A 38-year-old woman underwent Mohs surgery for in situ SCC arising in actinic keratosis on the left lateral upper eyelid and clinically involving the base of the lashes. The tumour-free defect measured 7 × 18 mm (**Photo A**).

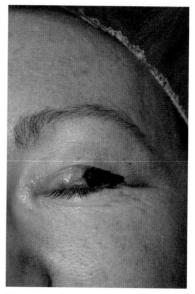

Photo A Left upper eyelid defect, post-Mohs surgery

Image courtesy of Duncan Stanford

QUESTION 1
What is your favoured repair option?

Answer
Full-thickness graft: A skin graft is generally best for the pre-tarsal component of both upper and lower eyelid defects; the entire defect in this case is pre-tarsal.

Comment on alternatives

In older patients, there may be sufficient skin to advance from above or lateral to the defect.

QUESTION 2

List suitable donor sites and discuss their relative merits.

Answer

1. Retroauricular skin
2. Preauricular skin
3. Upper eyelid

Retroauricular sulcus: The upper sulcus skin is suitably thin, easy to harvest and in an unobtrusive position, but is often pinker than the normal eyelid. The lower postauricular skin is generally a little thicker but may have a better colour match.

Preauricular skin: This skin is even easier to harvest but is slightly thicker than the postauricular skin and may be more suitable for lower eyelid and canthal defects.

Upper eyelid: Thin and matching skin is best harvested from this site but obtaining functionally and cosmetically pleasing results requires specific expertise. The donor site may be the same or opposite upper eyelid (**Photo B**). Possible issues include lid retraction, poor tapering above the lateral canthus and asymmetry. This younger woman does not have sufficient laxity in either eyelid.

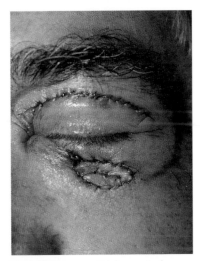

Photo B Upper eyelid donor site for lower eyelid graft in older man
Image courtesy of Duncan Stanford

QUESTION 3

Your oculoplastic colleague undertakes the repair, using lower retroauricular skin (**Photos C and D**). In **Photo C,** what is the long suture called, how is it inserted and what is the rationale for its use?

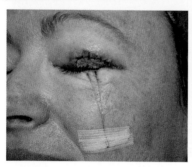 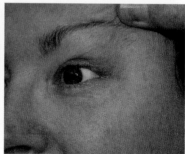

Photo C Full-thickness graft repair
Image courtesy of Duncan Stanford

Photo D Good outcome at 6 weeks.
Note permanent loss of eyelashes.
Image courtesy of Duncan Stanford

Answer

This traction suture has been inserted below the lower eyelid margin, out through its gray line, into the upper eyelid gray line, exited through the graft, been re-inserted back into the graft, exited the upper eyelid gray line, entered the lower eyelid gray line, then made a final exit through the lower eyelid skin below the lash line. The suture is left with long ends, which are taped to the upper cheek and left for 3–7 days.

The traction suture stabilises and immobilises the eyelid, enhancing graft take. Paraffin gauze and then double eye pads are applied for protection and pressure to further enhance graft take during this early operative period.

To remove the suture, one end is cut and the suture is gently pulled through and removed. Following traction suture removal, the eye is left open. The patient is requested to apply Chlorsig® or Refresh® eye ointment twice daily to the suture lines until complete healing occurs. The remainder of the sutures are removed at 7–10 days.

QUESTION 4

The patient returns to you during the second week post reconstruction, complaining of an itchy, swollen and irritated eye. She has been applying Chlorsig® ointment as directed by the oculoplastic surgeon. What diagnosis do you suspect and how would you confirm it?

Answer

Allergic contact dermatitis to chloramphenicol. (There is no preservative in the ointment preparation of chloramphenicol.) This is an uncommon problem and one should initially consider irritation from sutures (quite common) or infection.

A repeat open application test (ROAT) is a quick and easy way to assess for contact allergy. The ointment is applied to the same, small (at least 20 × 20 mm) and non-sun-exposed area of skin, twice daily for one week. Suitable areas for application include the flexor forearm, antecubital fossa, retroauricular area and lateral neck.

The reaction may be confirmed with formal patch testing.

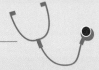

Section 7
Scalp

Case 27
Duncan Stanford and Shyamala Huilgol

A 66-year-old man presented with a moderately differentiated SCC on the frontal scalp (**Photo A**). The SCC was cleared by Mohs surgery in two stages, leaving a defect of 25 × 30 mm.

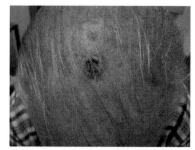

Photo A Scalp SCC
Image courtesy of Duncan Stanford

QUESTION 1
What technique is demonstrated in **Photo B** and how does it work?

Answer
Intra-operative photo shows pulley suture placed to achieve simple and inexpensive external tissue expansion while awaiting second and final frozen section pathology. This expansion works through tissue creep and stress relaxation. The sutures may be placed intra-operatively while awaiting Mohs sections or postoperatively before undertaking the repair.

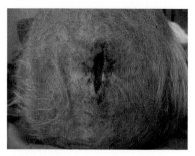

Photo B Pulley suture in place whilst awaiting final stage of Mohs pathology
Image courtesy of Duncan Stanford

These pulley sutures may also be left in place with long tails and then tightened weekly until primary closure is achieved.[1]

QUESTION 2
What three repair options would you consider?

Answer
1. Rotation flap
2. Split-thickness graft
3. Combined primary closure and central Burow's graft (**Photo C** and **Photo D**)

Comment on alternatives
Second intention healing can be an excellent alternative to split-thickness grafts on the scalp if sufficient tissue remains at the base. In this case, only periosteum remains so the outer table of the skull would need to be burred mechanically (e.g. with a bone saw). Healing is slow but gives a superior result compared to a split-thickness graft.

A bipedicle flap is another alternative; this could be unilateral but if insufficient movement is achieved, it could be converted to a bilateral flap.

Myocutaneous island pedicle flaps with lateral or inferior pedicles based on the frontalis are useful in the frontal scalp but may be technically challenging and are unlikely to be needed for this size of defect.

Full-thickness grafts to the entire defect are unlikely to take with only periosteum remaining at the base.

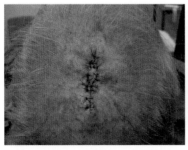

Photo C Combined primary closure and central Burow's graft
Image courtesy of Duncan Stanford

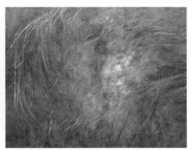

Photo D Outcome at 5 months
Image courtesy of Duncan Stanford

QUESTION 3

What are the advantages of Burow's full-thickness skin graft (FTSG) over FTSG to the entire defect?

Answer

Advantages

- The tissue match from this adjacent skin is often much better than from distant sites.
- Avoids second wound of donor site.
- Smaller graft means less metabolic demand, hence quicker and more reliable healing.
- Hair follicles preserved in hairy scalps.

Reference

1. Malone CH, McLaughlin JM, Ross LS et al. Progressive tightening of pulley sutures for primary repair of large scalp wounds. Plast Reconstr Surg Glob Open 2017 Dec; 5(12): e1592.

Case 28
Gilberto Moreno Bonilla and Shyamala Huilgol

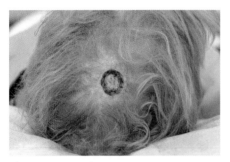

A 63-year-old woman had an infiltrating BCC on the scalp vertex treated with Mohs surgery. The tumour-free defect measured 21 × 23 mm (**Photo A**).

Photo A Post-Mohs surgery on vertex
Image courtesy of Gilberto Moreno Bonilla

QUESTION 1

Give your preferred closure option and two alternatives. Explain your reasoning.

Answer

Rotation flap

Alternatives:

1. Bridge flap
2. Second intention healing +/− partial closure
3. Split-thickness graft

Rotation flap: Local closures in hair-bearing skin give better outcomes than grafts. When primary closure is not possible, rotation flaps are the workhorse for medium to large scalp defects, offering a robust blood supply, relatively simple design and execution, and also the ability to cover areas of bare bone.

Bridge (bipedicle advancement) flaps are easily designed and redistribute tension away from the defect but generate less movement than rotation flaps. Usually single-sided, they may be converted to double-sided for added tissue movement.

Second intention healing requires vascularised tissue at the base and is useful where a flap closure is not possible or would be poorly tolerated, providing a better cosmetic outcome than a split-thickness graft, but at the cost of prolonged wound care. The eventual scar is half the defect size and level with the surrounding skin. Partial closure, including a purse string, may be used to reduce the defect size and healing time.

Split-thickness grafts are commonly used where the defect size is too great or unsuitable for local flap closure, including scarring from previous surgery. They are depressed, hairless, smooth and a different colour to the surrounding scalp but will take on a periosteum base.

Comment on alternatives

Full-thickness grafts may be used in small to medium defects with an intact galea and some subcutaneous tissue at the base. Excellent results may be obtained in hairless scalp or if a combination of partial closure and a hair-bearing Burow's graft are used. Transposition flaps are rarely used on their own by the authors on the scalp, excess tissue being more easily recruited with broad-based flaps. However, they are helpful in large defects when the secondary defect is repaired with a split-thickness graft.

QUESTION 2

Describe the design and execution of a scalp rotation flap with details on tissue depth and maximising cosmetic outcomes.

Answer

The standard scalp rotation flap design has a large arc from the edge of the defect in the direction of maximal tissue movement. Small flaps don't provide enough movement and are likely to fail due to the scalp's low elasticity and underlying, unyielding bone. The area under the arc is three to four times the defect size.

Incise the flap parallel to hair follicles (to prevent alopecia) and through the galea. Dissect and elevate the flap in the relatively avascular subgaleal plane.

After securing haemostasis, buried absorbable sutures approximate the galeal tissue to close the primary and then secondary defects. This prevents scar inversion and widening with noticeable alopecia. (An alternative approach is to undermine the flap and defect edges in a second, immediately supragaleal plane to free the sutured edges from downward tension, obviating the need for buried sutures. Avoid transecting hair bulbs to prevent alopecia.) Blanching of the sutured flap tip is not uncommon, but thanks to the large, broad-based pedicle, flap tip necrosis is rare. Excise the rotational pucker or dog ear. Interrupted superficial non-absorbable sutures or staples are used to gently approximate the skin edges (**Photos B** and **C**).

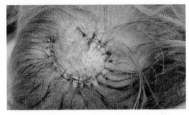 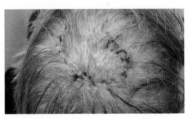

Photo B Standard rotation flap execution
Image courtesy of Gilberto Moreno Bonilla

Photo C Flap at 7 days
Image courtesy of Gilberto Moreno Bonilla

An alternative flap design commences with drawing a generous rotation flap dog ear at right angles to the direction of maximal movement. Usually, the defect is closed across its smallest axis, but if movement is clearly better in another direction, the defect may be closed across a wider point with an even longer dog ear.

Measure the radius from the point of rotation to the distal defect and draw an arc of rotation with an increasing radius to counter the expected loss of height during the rotational movement. (This loss of height creates the secondary crescent-shaped defect.) Additionally, as the underlying bone is both convex and incompressible, the radius needs to become progressively longer for the flap to go up and over the hard curved surface. Add 5 mm to the radius every 10–30 mm along the arc. In areas where the scalp is very convex (e.g. vertex) do so every 10–20 mm. If it is flatter (e.g. frontal scalp) make it every 20–30 mm. Join the series of dotted points into a large arc. Test the flap movement and remeasure the points and arc before proceeding (**Photos D** and **E**).

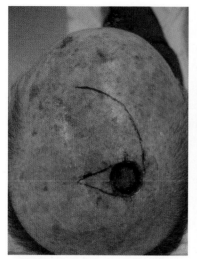

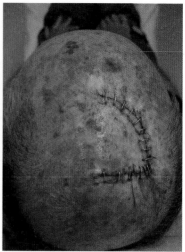

Photo D Modified scalp rotation flap design with increasing arc of rotation
Image courtesy of Shyamala Huilgol

Photo E Modified flap after closure
Image courtesy of Shyamala Huilgol

QUESTION 3
Discuss options when the flap is under excessive tension.

Answer

In cases with excessive tension, options include placing pulley sutures and waiting for tissue creep and stress relaxation; adding a Burow's triangle (anywhere external to the arc but often at its end); adding a back-cut to the flap; converting to a double rotation flap; and closing the primary defect while grafting the secondary defect. Galeotomy incisions in the tissue surrounding the flap and parallel to the wound edge permit extra secondary tissue movement.

Double rotation flap of O–Z design introduce additional scars, greater complexity and tissue manipulation, and a higher risk of flap tip necrosis. If the dog ear has not already been removed, this repair can salvage a single rotation flap that is unable to close the defect or is under too much tension. Double rotation flaps of "anchor" design do not provide as much tissue movement but may be used where the dog ear has been removed.

QUESTION 4

The patient returned at 7 days (**Photo C**) for suture removal, reporting intense pain on days 1 and 2. What pain management is recommended after skin surgery?

Answer

The patient should be reassured there is no evidence of infection, haematoma or flap necrosis. Few prospective studies are available regarding postoperative pain and relief. Most patients obtain pain control with simple analgesia (paracetamol with or without ibuprofen).[1] A small minority require opioids (paracetamol with codeine) in the first 36 hours. Management of pre- and intra-operative anxiety decreases pain. Risk factors for greater postoperative pain include flap or graft repair; scalp, lip, ear or nose location; young age; and an increased number of treated sites. Injecting plain 0.5% bupivacaine HCl after flap reconstruction decreased pain and the need for opioid analgesia in a prospective, placebo-controlled trial.[2]

References

1. Sniezek P, Brodland D, Zitelli J. A randomized controlled trial comparing acetaminophen, acetaminophen and ibuprofen, and acetaminophen and codeine for postoperative pain relief after Mohs surgery and cutaneous reconstruction. Dermatol Surg 2011; 37(7): 1007–1013.
2. Voss V, Oh C, Veerabagu S, Nugent S, Giordano C, Golda N. Bupivacaine to reduce pain and narcotic use after Mohs micrographic surgery. Dermatol Surg 2022; 48(11): 1135–1139.

Section 8
Neck and mastoid

Case 29
Shyamala Huilgol and Duncan Stanford

A 60-year-old man presented with a recurrent nodular BCC in the right mastoid area after two previous excisions by his skin cancer clinic doctor. The tumour was cleared in two Mohs surgery stages, with a final defect of 28 × 43 mm (**Photo A**).

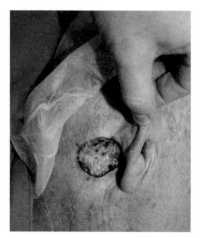

Photo A Post-Mohs surgery defect centred over right mastoid
Image courtesy of Duncan Stanford

QUESTION 1
What are your three favoured repair options? Comment on their relative merits.

Answer
1. Transposition flap
2. Advancement flap
3. Split-thickness graft

Comment
The lax skin in the lateral neck is both inferior and posterior to this defect. This laxity may be recruited with a transposition flap, altering

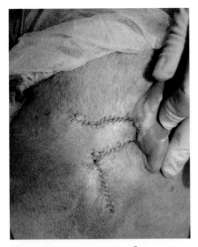

Photo B Post-transposition flap repair
Image courtesy of Duncan Stanford

the direction and aligning the secondary defect closure within the natural neck creases (**Photo B**).

An advancement flap would recruit skin in a more straightforward fashion: the long arm of the flap would extend along the postauricular sulcus and inferiorly onto the lateral neck, following the natural neck creases with the dog ear or Burow's triangle extending posteriorly behind the defect.

A split-thickness graft would be possible; the poorer cosmetic outcome will have less impact in this partially hidden site.

Comment on alternatives

Primary closure is not possible. A full-thickness graft might not take, given that this location is subject to tension each time the head is turned. Second intention healing would be possible.

QUESTION 2

A transposition flap is performed. What concerns do you have looking at the repair in **Photo B**?

Answer

The flap is blanched, suggesting some compromise of the blood supply. This may lead to flap tip necrosis and subsequent distortion of the ear position if left to heal by second intention.

QUESTION 3

What easy manoeuvre could you to do to assess and relieve vascular compromise?

Answer

Place the ear back in its normal position to relieve tension arising from pulling it forwards and reassess the flap colour after a few minutes.

In this case, the flap colour returned to normal with a good long-term result (**Photo C**).

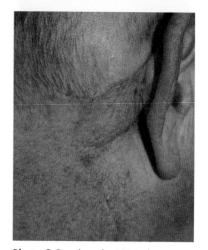

Photo C Good result at 6 weeks postop. The ear position is normal with no pinning back. Note that geometric scar lines are highlighted by scar erythema which is likely to fade, and the colour discrepancy due to the donor site being more sun damaged than the postauricular area. Both of these were inconsequential to patient given the location.

Image courtesy of Duncan Stanford

QUESTION 4

Is there anything that you could do to improve blood flow and outcomes if the flap remains blanched with the ear in this normal anatomic position?

Answer

Sometimes a flap will blanch as buried sutures are placed. This may be due to a key vessel being compromised as well as the usual problem of excessive tension. If this happens, remove this suture and try re-suturing in a different position. If blanching only occurred after cutaneous sutures were placed, consider removing them and re-suturing. This is easier if interrupted cutaneous sutures have been used: one or a few can be easily removed to assess whether removing focal tension leads to pinking of the flap. If so, it may be reasonable to leave an area unsutured and permit second intention healing in this focal area.

Commonly, blanching is due to excessive tension with the flap being overly stretched. The flap's design and motion may need to be altered; it is always better to do so at this point rather than waiting for flap necrosis to develop. Further undermining of the pivot point in this flap might assist with its transposition into the defect. Reducing the effective defect size can help an otherwise too small flap become sufficient for the job. An offcut can be used as a Burow's graft to a portion of the defect or the defect's size can be reduced by removing a dog ear from a favourable point (e.g. the retroauricular sulcus).

(This flap is not amenable to major reworking, but other flaps may respond to measures including extending the arc of rotation, lengthening a dog ear or altering the angle of closure of the secondary defect.)

If you are happy with the flap's design and suturing and believe that the problem is temporary, the routine use of hourly cold packs for 10–15 minutes on the day of surgery may be extended into the following day. This will lower the flap's metabolic demand and postoperative swelling, both factors helping to salvage the flap.

The dressing may be used to reduce tension on the flap—using strong adhesive, non-woven fabric tape such as Hypafix® to lift and support the flap movement.

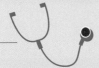

Section 9
Trunk and limbs

Case 30
Shyamala Huilgol and Duncan Stanford

A 74-year-old man presented with a rapidly recurring SCC on the dorsum of the left hand after incomplete excision two months previously. The pathology report showed a well-differentiated SCC extending to both lateral margins and 2 mm clear of the deep margin. There was no perineural or intravascular invasion. The depth and level of invasion were not reported. The tumour was 20 mm in diameter (**Photo A**).

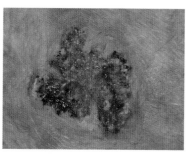

Photo A Preoperative view of the hand SCC

Image courtesy of Duncan Stanford

QUESTION 1
What two clinical findings should you assess?

Answer
The tumour was not attached to underlying tendons, moving freely over these. There was no palpable lymphadenopathy in the epitrochlear, axillary and cervical lymph nodes.

QUESTION 2
The tumour was cleared with one Mohs surgery stage, resulting in a defect of 40 × 50 mm (**Photo B**). List three repair options you would consider for this defect.

Answer
1. Full-thickness graft

2. Partial closure with either central full-thickness graft or second intention healing
3. Second intention healing

Comment on alternatives
The defect is too large for a transposition flap. A split-thickness graft will not provide durability for the hand location. Primary closure is not possible.

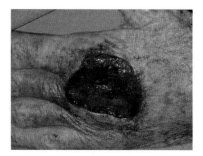

Photo B Post-Mohs surgery defect
Image courtesy of Duncan Stanford

QUESTION 3
You decide to do a full-thickness skin graft. List three potential donor sites.

Answer
1. Flexor surface of forearm
2. Upper inner arm
3. Clavicle

QUESTION 4
Describe your technique for a full-thickness skin graft.

Answer
1. Choose donor site: the ipsilateral forearm is chosen for the good colour and texture match as well as a width of 40+ mm available skin.
2. Make a template of the defect from a non-adherent dressing (e.g. Telfa®).
3. After cleansing the donor site with an alcohol swab, the template is placed with the long axis along the forearm's natural diagonal skin creases. The marked size of the required donor skin is oversized by 5 mm to allow for shrinkage after harvesting, as this site is usually under tension. Triangular dog ears are added to the oval to form an ellipse aligned in the skin creases.
4. Local anaesthetic is infiltrated into the donor and recipient sites.

5. Using sterile technique, the graft is harvested with a combination of initial scalpel incision of the lateral edges to the subcutaneous tissue and blunt scissor excision at the depth, taking care to maintain the same depth through subcutaneous tissue. The graft is placed in sterile normal saline after harvesting. It is optional to fenestrate the graft before or after harvesting. The donor wound edges are undermined approx. 5 mm to enhance closure and improve scar quality. Electrosurgical haemostasis to the donor site is carried out. The wound is closed with a layered closure with 4-0 buried interrupted absorbable sutures (e.g. polyglecaprone) and 4-0 cutaneous non-absorbable sutures (e.g. nylon).

6. The recipient site is inspected and treated to ensure adequate haemostasis. The graft is lightly defatted and placed on the defect, and then moved with forceps so that the two lateral sides approximate the defect edges. An interrupted cutaneous 5-0 silk suture is used to hold each of these opposing sides of the graft in position. All sutures are placed from the graft to the recipient edge ("ship to shore"). One of the longer poles of the donor ellipse is trimmed to fit into the third side of the defect and sutured into place. Lastly, the remaining long pole is trimmed to fit the defect and another interrupted suture placed. All edges of the graft are assessed and trimmed as needed before using further interrupted or running sutures to hold the graft in place (**Photo C**).

Comment

Nylon, polypropylene or absorbable polyglactin 910 (Vicryl Rapide®) sutures are good alternatives. No bolster is usually used in this site, but it would be reasonable to do so. In this site with underlying tendons, pexing sutures through the base of the graft and fenestration of the graft *in situ* are not recommended.

QUESTION 5

What postoperative care would you arrange?

Answer

Dressing: A non-adherent dressing (e.g. Melolin®) is cut slightly larger than the graft, coated in white soft petrolatum and applied to the graft. A second, slightly larger piece of the dressing is applied, and then adhesive, non-woven fabric tape (e.g. Hypafix®) used to hold both layers in place. Soft rayon fleece orthopaedic padding (e.g. Soffban®) is wrapped around the hand and wrist as a first layer, followed by 2–3 layers of self-adherent elastic wrap (e.g. Coban®) and the hand is placed in a collar and cuff sling. Aftercare: The patient is asked to keep the dressing dry and intact until suture removal, to limit physical activity and keep the hand elevated in the sling during the day but is permitted to remove the sling at night and for small and gentle tasks like eating. The patient may completely remove the Coban® if it feels too tight and reapply it more loosely.

These instructions are given in writing along with after- and in-hours contact details in case of postoperative problems, including infection, bleeding and pain.

Medications: Cephalexin 1 g one hour preoperatively followed by 500 mg qid are prescribed for 5 days. Paracetamol 500–1000 mg prn (max. 4 g/24 hours) is suggested for postoperative pain relief.

Appointments: Removal of sutures for both donor and graft is booked for 10–14 days. After suture removal, the patient is asked to apply post-shower daily dressings to the graft with white soft petrolatum, a non-stick dressing (e.g. Melolin®) and tape for a further week. Hypafix® is applied to the donor site and left *in situ* for a further week. After showering, the patient should dry the tape with a towel or hair dryer.

The graft had good vascularisation at removal of sutures 12 days postop (**Photo D**), and at 2-month follow-up had completely taken with very good tissue match.

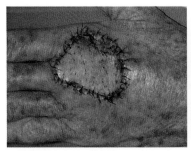

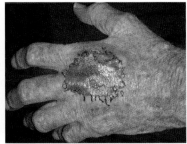

Photo C Graft sutured in place with 4-0 interrupted silk sutures
Image courtesy of Duncan Stanford

Photo D Graft at suture removal, 12 days postop. Note healthy pink colour with complete take of the graft.
Image courtesy of Duncan Stanford

Case 31
Shyamala Huilgol

A 74-year-old man presented with a biopsy-proven, superficial and infiltrating BCC on the right lateral lower leg, measuring 15 × 15 mm **(Photo A)**.

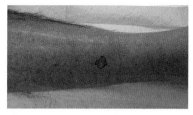

Photo A BCC on the right lower leg
Image courtesy of Shyamala Huilgol

QUESTION 1
List treatment options for this tumour.

Answer
1. Standard excision with 4–5 mm margins
2. Mohs surgery excision to ensure complete excision and minimise tissue loss

Comment on alternatives
Radiotherapy is relatively contraindicated on the lower leg with its potential for poor wound healing and chronic ulceration. Topical 5-fluorouracil, imiquimod and photodynamic therapy are not recommended with infiltrating BCC histology.

QUESTION 2

The patient undergoes Mohs surgery, resulting in a 17 × 20 mm tumour-free defect (**Photo B**). List reconstructive options in order of preference and discuss their relative merits.

Answer

1. Keystone island flap
2. Split-thickness graft
3. Partial primary closure with Burow's graft
4. Full-thickness graft
5. Subcutaneous island pedicle flap/s
6. Bipedicle (bridge) flap

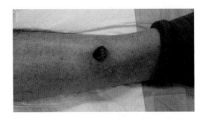

Photo B Post-Mohs surgery lower leg defect

Image courtesy of Shyamala Huilgol

Comment

The lower limb is a difficult surgical site, often hampered by venous, lymphatic and arterial compromise and practical difficulties in immobilisation.

Flaps heal more quickly, preserve contour and look better than split-thickness grafts. However, oedema may occur, despite efforts to preserve blood vessels, and they cannot be performed directly over the shin. The keystone island flap is the workhorse flap repair on the lower leg, with ease of execution and reliable healing, even in scarred and irradiated tissue.

Split-thickness grafts are the usual alternative but often suffer partial failure, being susceptible to movement, fluid drainage and infection. Full-thickness grafts are more robust and offer better cosmesis, but need good vascularity. A degree of second intention healing may be needed in both grafts. Grafts require a donor site. The split-thickness donor site may be painful and very slow to heal, usually resulting in a pale rectangular scar. Partial primary closure with use of the dog ear as a Burow's graft is a simpler procedure for smaller defects and avoids a donor site. Subcutaneous island flaps are prone to trapdooring and may be surprisingly difficult to mobilise; using everting sutures and two opposing flaps may help. Bipedicle flaps are useful but blind undermining may damage deep blood vessels.

Comment on alternatives

Primary closure alone is not possible. Transposition and rotation flaps are difficult to mobilise and less reliable.

QUESTION 3

Describe the design and execution of a classic keystone flap and possible modifications.

Answer

Design: The defect is converted into an ellipse, parallel to blood vessels and nerves to reduce potential damage. The classic design is a curved trapezoid, parallel to the primary elliptical defect in an area of greater laxity, the flap width being at least equal to the defect width (**Photo C**).[1] To facilitate closure, one may round off the two projections of the flap's advancing margin, increase the angle of the flap to more than 90° and elongate the two apices (**Photo D**). Variations include double keystone flaps and partial incision of the flap margins. Doppler mapping of flap perforators may help avoid damage.

Execution: Under sterile conditions, incise the flap down to the fascia, then undermine primary and secondary defects, leaving larger blood vessels intact during incision and undermining. Obtain haemostasis, suturing larger vessels as needed. Advance the flap into the defect with 1 to 3 buried absorbable key sutures (3-0 or 4-0 poliglecaprone 25 or polyglactin 910), use further buried sutures for

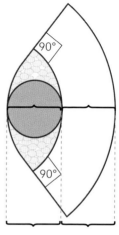

$$\frac{\text{Exisional width}}{} = \frac{\text{Flap width}}{}$$

Ratio at least 1:1

Photo C Classic keystone flap

Source: Stanford D, Storey L. Dermatologic Surgery: A manual of defect repairs options. 2nd ed. Australia: McGraw Hill 2023.

double V–Y closure of the upper and lower apices, then close remainder of flap. Buried Haneke–Marini and inverted cross mattress sutures may assist with tension.[2,3] Use staples and/or cutaneous sutures (4-0 nylon) for skin closure (**Photo E**). Pulley or mattress sutures with 3-0 or 4-0 nylon are helpful to close the flap and evert edges while staples are placed and may then be removed. Apply non-stick dressing for 48 hours and change daily after showering. Use T.E.D.™ stockings (15–20 mm Hg) during the day with constant leg elevation and limit walking to toilet privileges only. Remove staples/sutures at 2–3 weeks, then support wound with Hypafix® tape and ongoing T.E.D.™ stockings for a further 2–3 weeks. Oral antibiotics should be considered at this site, especially in those with co-existing morbidities. The long-term outcome is shown in **Photo F.**

If there are difficulties in mobilising the flap, the deep fascia on the side of the flap furthest from the defect may be incised, released and incorporated into the flap. In those with thin skin, placing deep sutures may prove impossible. Cutaneous sutures alone may be used and left for 4–5 weeks. If the skin tears with placement of cutaneous sutures, sterile Hypafix may be applied to strengthen the edges of the wound and staples/sutures placed through the tape (**Photo G**).

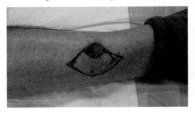

Photo D Keystone flap plan showing standard markings and amended design. Note flap width increased from initial markings to be greater than defect width, increase in flap angle from initial 90° to more than 90° and elongation of flap apices to reduce V–Y angle of closure.

Image courtesy of Shyamala Huilgol

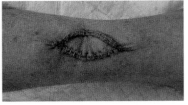

Photo E Flap closure. Note excision of two leading points of flap during closure.

Image courtesy of Shyamala Huilgol

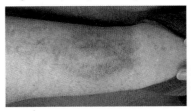

Photo F Long-term outcome at 3 months. Note hyperpigmentation from co-existent venous disease.

Image courtesy of Shyamala Huilgol

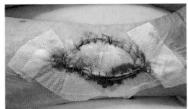

Photo G Hypafix used to support thin skin and permit cutaneous closure in a different patient

Image courtesy of Shyamala Huilgol

QUESTION 4

Describe your execution of a split-thickness graft to the lower leg.

Answer

Measure the defect, add a 1 cm margin of safety to the length and width. Mark this rectangle on the ipsilateral anterior thigh. Administer local anaesthesia proximally, wait some minutes (nerves travel proximally to distally), then inject remainder of the periphery and centrally. Top up the primary defect. Ropivacaine 0.75% with 1:200,000 adrenaline provides less pain, greater diffusion and reduced adrenaline side effects.

Using sterile technique, ask your assistant to apply traction with two handheld sterile boards and use either a handheld knife dermatome (e.g. Weck, Silvers) or electric/air dermatome (e.g. Zimmer®) to harvest the graft. Place graft on the defect (after haemostasis) or into normal saline. Apply saline-soaked or 3% hydrogen peroxide-soaked gauze to the donor site. Consider graft fenestration (lift and incise with fine scissors), then trim to 3 mm larger than defect. Use tissue glue (e.g. Dermabond®) or fast-absorbing 6-0 sutures (e.g. Vicryl rapide™) on graft edges. Prevent glue from running into the wound as healing will be impaired. Central basting sutures are usually unnecessary. Apply slightly oversized, non-stick mesh layer (e.g. Adaptic™) and then three ovals of absorptive foam bolster (e.g. Allevyn), the smaller two sized to sit inside the graft margins, and press it into the defect with the larger to sit 10–15 mm outside the graft (**Photo H**). Use staples to hold the larger piece of foam to the skin outside the graft and centrally to hold the foam layers together. Avoid using petrolatum jelly or paraffin gauze with tissue glue as it will dissolve it. One may also use a variety of tied bolster techniques. T.E.D.™ stockings and restriction of activity were previously described.

On the donor site, the dressing options include weekly foam dressing (e.g. Allevyn™). The graft bolster is removed at 2 weeks and ongoing daily petrolatum jelly, non-stick dressings, tape and T.E.D.™ stockings are applied to graft and donor until healing is complete. Weekly wound review in clinic until healing is complete is helpful.

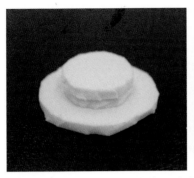
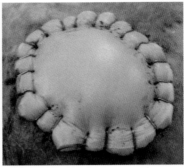

Photo H Inverted wedding cake foam bolster with staples
Source: Stanford D, Storey L. Dermatologic Surgery: A manual of defect repairs options.
2nd ed. Australia: McGraw Hill 2023.

References

1. Behan FC. The keystone design perforator island flap in reconstructive surgery. ANZ J Surg 2003; 73: 112–20.
2. Marini L. The Haneke-Marini suture: not a "new" technique. Dermatol Surg 1995; 21: 819–20.
3. Yag-Howard C. Novel surgical approach to subcutaneous closure: the subcutaneous inverted cross mattress stitch (SICM stitch). Dermatol Surg 2011; 31: 1503–5.

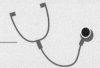

Section 10
Multidisciplinary cases

Case 32.1
Jessica Tong, Shyamala Huilgol and Dinesh Selva

A 65-year-old man with a small BCC on his right central lower eyelid (**Photo A**) undergoes Mohs surgery, resulting in a 10-mm defect (**Photo B**).

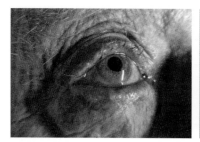

Photo A BCC on right eyelid
Image courtesy of Dinesh Selva

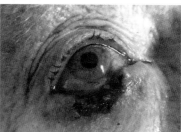

Photo B Post-Mohs surgery lower lid defect with edges freshened and sharpened prior to closure
Image courtesy of Dinesh Selva

QUESTION 1
How could this defect (**Photo B**) be repaired?

Answer

A small full-thickness eyelid defect is usually managed with a wedge excision and primary closure.

This defect could be left to heal by secondary intention. This will take some weeks and require supervision, with the potential for suboptimal functional and cosmetic outcomes including a notch, poor lid contour or cicatricial lower lid ectropion.

QUESTION 2

Outline the steps in wedge excision and primary closure.

Answer

The defect is first converted into a pentagon (**Photo B**). The tarsus is directly closed with two 6-0 absorbable sutures (e.g. Vicryl®), ensuring that there is a smooth lid margin contour with no step. Further buried sutures are placed, one in the gray line for marginal closure, then others to close the orbicularis and then the skin. The skin is then closed with 6-0 short-acting absorbable sutures (e.g. Vicryl rapide®). Early follow-up is shown in **Photo C.**

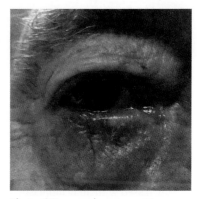

Photo C Two-week postoperative appearance with good eyelid contour
Image courtesy of Dinesh Selva

Case 32.2
Jessica Tong, Shyamala Huilgol and Dinesh Selva

A 78-year-old man undergoes Mohs surgery for a left lower eyelid infiltrating BCC, resulting in a 7 × 15 mm defect (**Photo D**). You have already liaised with an oculoplastic surgeon to perform the repair.

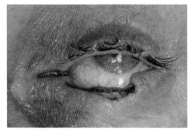

Photo D Post-Mohs surgery defect of the left lower lid
Image courtesy of Dinesh Selva

QUESTION 3
What is an appropriate reconstruction method for this medium-sized, full-thickness eyelid defect?

Answer
Tenzel semicircular flaps are used for lower lid defects that cannot be closed directly with a wedge repair and measure 15 mm or less when approximated under tension. There must be sufficient lateral lid remaining to be advanced medially for defect closure.

Alternative bilamellar closures are discussed in the next case (Case 32.3).

QUESTION 4

Describe a Tenzel flap reconstruction to a junior colleague.

Answer

1. A shallow curve is marked, originating at the lateral canthus (**Photo E**).
2. The skin and orbicularis flap is raised (**Photo F**) with a lateral canthotomy and inferior cantholysis (**Photo G**). Beyond the lateral orbital rim, the flap depth becomes more superficial — within subcutaneous fat — to prevent injury to the temporal branch of the facial nerve lying within the superficial temporal fascia.
3. As the lateral lid remnant and Tenzel flap are mobilised medially, the flap is widely undermined with a titrated release of the tarsus from the conjunctiva-retractor complex to enable defect closure (**Photo H**).
4. The primary defect is closed, using two 6-0 absorbable sutures (e.g. Vicryl) to appose the tarsus, followed by a marginal suture at the gray line (**Photo I**).
5. The Tenzel flap is anchored to the periosteum above the lateral canthal tendon attachment with a 4-0 long-acting absorbable suture (e.g. Vicryl). This suture provides crucial vertical support at the lateral canthus to prevent lower lid retraction (**Photo J**).
6. Finally, the lateral canthal angle is re-formed with absorbable sutures and the skin is closed (**Photo K**).

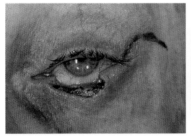 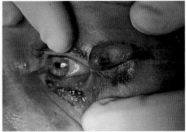

Photo E A shallow curve is marked at the lateral canthus
Image courtesy of Dinesh Selva

Photo F The skin and orbicularis flap with lateral dissection within the subcutaneous fat
Image courtesy of Dinesh Selva

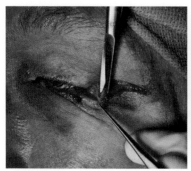

Photo G An inferior cantholysis frees the skin-orbicularis flap
Image courtesy of Dinesh Selva

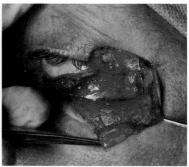

Photo H Tarsal release from the conjunctiva and lower lid retractors with sub-orbicularis dissection to mobilise flap
Image courtesy of Dinesh Selva

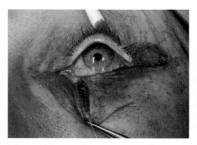

Photo I Marginal suture at gray line closes the primary defect
Image courtesy of Dinesh Selva

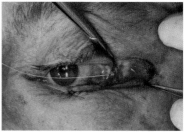

Photo J The Tenzel flap is anchored onto the periosteum above the lateral canthal tendon
Image courtesy of Dinesh Selva

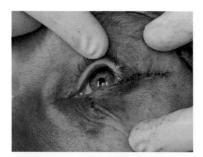

Photo K Immediate postoperative appearance. The lower lid is well-apposed to the globe and the lateral canthal angle has been reformed.
Image courtesy of Dinesh Selva

Case 32.3
Jessica Tong, Shyamala Huilgol and Dinesh Selva

A 74-year-old man undergoes Mohs surgery excision of an extensive eyelid BCC, with removal of nearly the entire lower eyelid (**Photo L**). Preoperatively, you have liaised with an oculoplastic surgeon who will reconstruct the defect.

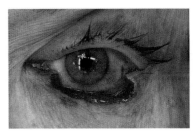

Photo L Extensive lower lid defect
Image courtesy of Dinesh Selva

QUESTION 5
Discuss reconstruction options for this complex defect.

Answer

This large defect requires a bilamellar reconstruction to replace the two layers of mucosa/tarsus and skin. This can be achieved with either a lid-sharing pedicled (Hughes) flap or graft combined with a skin flap.

The Hughes flap uses the superior half of the upper eyelid tarsus supported by a conjunctival pedicle to re-create the posterior lamella, combined with a full-thickness skin graft or local flap for the anterior lamella. A skin graft can be sourced from the upper lid, preauricular, postauricular, supraclavicular or inner brachial regions. During the 1–2 week phase with the pedicle, the eye is initially patched and then left open. The second stage of the procedure involves division of the conjunctival pedicle with establishment of a new lower lid margin.

Alternatively, a posterior lamellar graft may be combined with an anterior lamellar flap to support the graft, particularly in monocular patients who would be unable to have their sole eye unusable during a pedicled flap. The posterior lamella graft must have both sufficient rigidity and a mucosal lining, best found with a contralateral tarsal graft. Other donor options include hard palate mucosa, nasal septal cartilage with mucoperichondrium, auricular cartilage, buccal or labial mucosa, although the latter two will likely have insufficient rigidity.

QUESTION 6
Describe a Hughes flap reconstruction to a junior colleague.

Answer

1. The horizontal dimension of the lower lid defect is measured with the defect opposed as much as possible (i.e. under tension) to determine the flap width.

2. A traction suture is placed through the upper lid margin, which is everted on a Desmarres retractor.

3. Four millimetres of residual tarsus is preserved adjacent to the lid margin, to prevent entropion of the upper lid. This 4 mm margin is marked, along with the required flap width.

4. The flap is incised through the tarsus, parallel to the lid margin, and vertical cuts are made upwards and towards the conjunctiva. The pedicle can be dissected to contain Müller's muscle and conjunctiva (**Photo M**) or conjunctiva alone (**Photo N**).

5. The flap is sutured into the defect with 6-0 long-acting absorbable sutures (e.g. Vicryl). Flap inset is crucial in determining lid margin contour. The tarsal flap must be parallel with the lid remnants or slightly proud, which can be adjusted at the second stage. For a lower lid defect without lateral support, an additional periosteal flap may be transposed from the lateral orbital rim.

6. The anterior surface of the tarsus is covered with a full-thickness skin graft or local flap. A graft should be placed 1–2 mm inferior to the new lid margin (**Photo O**).

7. The conjunctival pedicle can be divided after 1–2 weeks. The new lower lid margin is sculpted flush with the adjacent tarsal segments and left to heal by secondary intention. Müller's muscle is recessed from the conjunctival pedicle to prevent future lid retraction. The amount of recession is titrated according to the upper lid contour and height. The upper tarsoconjunctival defect is left to granulate (**Photo P**).

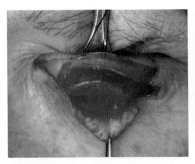

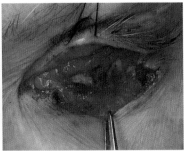

Photo M The upper lid is everted with 4 mm of preserved tarsus adjacent to the lid margin. The tarsoconjunctival flap is separated from the orbital septum. Müller's muscle remains on the conjunctiva. The retractor is visible through the anterior lamella.
Image courtesy of Dinesh Selva

Photo N Müller's muscle is recessed from the conjunctiva, freeing the tarsoconjunctival flap
Image courtesy of Dinesh Selva

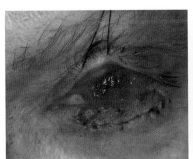

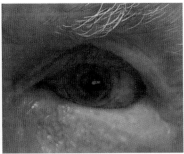

Photo O A Hughes flap with overlying skin graft. The cornea is visible underneath the thin conjunctiva.
Image courtesy of Dinesh Selva

Photo P One year following Hughes flap reconstruction, with lower lid well-apposed to the globe and normal upper lid contour
Image courtesy of Dinesh Selva

QUESTION 7

What are the specific complications of complex eyelid reconstructions with Tenzel and Hughes flaps?

Answer

- **Tenzel:** Poor lid contour with concavity at the site of primary closure; lower lid retraction; lateral canthus rounding or conjunctival granuloma formation; wound dehiscence.
- **Hughes:** Upper or lower lid retraction; lash ptosis; lower lid margin issues — prolonged erythema and thickening, ectropion or entropion **(Photos Q** and **R).**

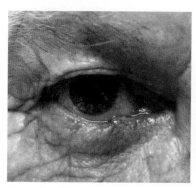 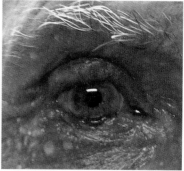

Photo Q Mild lower lid retraction following Hughes flap
Image courtesy of Dinesh Selva

Photo R Upper lid lash ptosis, upper eyelid retraction and lower lid margin erythema following Hughes flap
Image courtesy of Dinesh Selva

Reference

1. Collin JRO. A Manual of Systematic Eyelid Surgery. 3rd ed. Butterworth-Heinemann; 2005.

Case 33
Gilberto Moreno Bonilla and Shyamala Huilgol

An otherwise well 93-year-old man presented with two new lesions on the right scalp vertex and the right mandibular cheek, 11 months after excision and split-thickness grafting of an SCC on the scalp vertex (**Photos A and B**).

QUESTION 1
Outline your approach, including further investigations.

Answer

Clinical examination: New lesions on the same side as the previously excised cutaneous SCC (cSCC) raise the possibility of recurrence and locoregional disease spread or in-transit metastasis. The new scalp tumour arose directly adjacent to the graft, suggesting recurrence. The SCC on the right mandibular cheek lay within the draining lymphatics over the

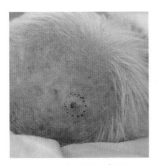

Photo A Scalp SCC of 20 mm diameter, adjacent to previous graft
Image courtesy of Gilberto Moreno Bonilla

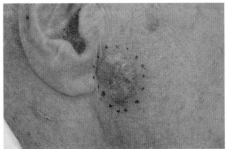

Photo B New SCC 30 mm in diameter on the right cheek
Image courtesy of Gilberto Moreno Bonilla

parotid, raising the possibility of in-transit metastasis. Cervical lymph node palpation for metastases was unremarkable. Targeted cranial nerve examination for sensation and motor function was normal.

Pathology: The previous pathology should be reviewed. The original lesion had been 40 mm in diameter and was reported as poorly differentiated, invading to 8.3 mm depth into subcutaneous fat, with clearance of 1.2 mm at the depth and 3 mm at peripheral margins. Immediate punch or incisional biopsy is required of both lesions to assess prognostic factors and exclude in-transit metastasis.

Staging: An urgent contrast CT scan of head and neck will assess bone integrity, the parotid gland and cervical lymph nodes. A PET CT scan to rule out distant metastasis may also be considered. It's important to assess renal function (especially at the patient's age) and any medications affecting kidney function prior to organising a contrast scan. The role of sentinel lymph node biopsy in high-risk cSCC remains undefined, with no clear survival benefit identified. A number of prognostic biomarker and genetic tumour profiling tests are under investigation, with their role yet to be clarified.

Treatment: Urgent Mohs surgery is indicated if CT scanning excludes metastases; higher cure rates being achieved from complete margin assessment.[1] Formal pathology staging of the centrally debulked tumour with paraffin sections is helpful in both risk factor assessment and subsequent communication with colleagues. Any clinical suspicion or histological (frozen or paraffin sections) findings of significant perineural invasion (PNI) should prompt consideration of an MRI neurographic protocol with neuroradiologist review to exclude large nerve PNI. Adjuvant postoperative radiotherapy and multidisciplinary team (MDT) review should also be considered given the high-risk nature of both tumours.

QUESTION 2
Define high-risk cSCC, including prognostic factors. Which one currently appears to be the most important?

Answer
High-risk cSCC has a higher risk of poor outcomes, including tumour recurrence, metastasis and disease-specific death. A 5% or greater risk of lymph node metastasis may be used as a helpful defining feature.

High-risk tumours need ongoing surveillance, nodal evaluation and consideration of adjuvant multimodal treatment so their initial identification through staging is important. The most widely used cSCC staging systems are AJCC-8[2] and BWH[3] but their ability to correctly predict bad outcomes is somewhat limited, with 30% of metastatic SCC not identified as higher risk.[4] These staging systems rely upon assessment of tumour, draining nodes and distant metastases (TNM staging). In clinical practice, most SCCs have neither nodal nor distant metastases, hence the focus is on assessment of the tumour itself. Both staging systems rely upon tumour size and depth, and the presence of deeper or larger nerve PNI; while BWH also adds poor differentiation. The development of staging systems predicting risks of local recurrence, metastasis and disease-specific death, as well as the assessment of treatment efficacy, have been hampered by different study designs and cohorts, a lack of uniform pathology reporting and varying treatment regimens.

A systematic review and meta-analysis[5] found depth of tumour invasion—measured in millimetres or anatomically—to be the most relevant factor in predicting poor outcomes, including local recurrence and nodal metastasis. However, accurate measurement, compromised by shave or incomplete biopsies, and inconsistent reporting limit its value.

In clinical practice, the authors have found the National Comprehensive Cancer Network (NCCN) guidelines helpful in identifying other high-risk features for consideration, including higher risk locations (head, neck, hands, feet, pretibial and anogenital), poor definition, recurrence, immunosuppression, previous radiation or chronic inflammation, rapid growth, neurologic symptoms, higher risk histological features (acantholytic, adenosquamoid and metaplastic subtypes) and lymphovascular invasion (LVI). Other factors with independent associations with poor outcomes include increased age, high tumour budding and ulceration. Other staging systems and guidelines include those developed by Breuninger, the Union for International Cancer Control and the European Interdisciplinary Guidelines.

QUESTION 3

Both biopsies showed epidermal origin of poorly differentiated cSCC, at least 4.5 mm in Breslow depth, with no PNI/LVI or features of in-transit metastasis. Kidney function was normal, and a contrast CT scan of head and neck showed no abnormalities in lymph nodes, soft tissues or bone. Mohs surgery was performed at both sites. The scalp lesion was cleared in one stage with a final defect of 30 × 35 mm. The right cheek sections demonstrated incidental PNI in an extra-tumoral nerve of <0.1 mm diameter, 0.6 mm from the margin, requiring a second stage with a final defect size of 33 × 39 mm (**Photo C**). Briefly describe closure options at both sites and further management.

Answer

Both sites require ongoing monitoring for local recurrence, hence closures should minimise tissue rearrangement. The scalp defect would benefit from a full- or split-thickness skin graft (**Photo D**), permitting easy monitoring for local recurrence without distortion from a flap. However, if adjuvant radiotherapy is being considered, a more durable flap would be preferable to prevent post-radiation ulceration and osteonecrosis.

The cheek defect could be simply closed with a tripolar advancement flap (limbs in front and behind ear and along jawline); a combination of partial closure and grafting or second intention healing; or a Limberg

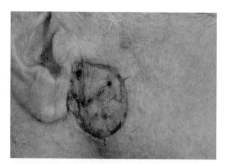

Photo C Right cheek post-Mohs surgery defect

Image courtesy of Gilberto Moreno Bonilla

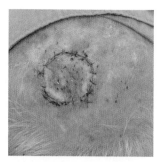

Photo D Right scalp vertex following full-thickness skin graft repair

Image courtesy of Gilberto Moreno Bonilla

rhombic flap from the infra-auricular skin. The first two have the benefit of minimising tissue rearrangement but are likely to be less cosmetically pleasing than the rhombic flap.

Given the number of high-risk features, MDT assessment at a tertiary centre is recommended. Adjuvant radiotherapy to primary sites and draining lymph nodes should be considered for these high-risk tumours, albeit tempered by the patient's advanced age. In addition to age, patient preference, comorbidities and ECOG performance status (a measure of functioning in daily living activities) are important in assessment of suitability for additional radiation and systemic treatment.

While PNI with clinical symptoms or detected on MRI has a clearly increased risk of adverse outcomes and warrants consideration of adjuvant radiotherapy, adjuvant radiotherapy for lesser degrees of PNI (as in this case) is individually assessed. A recent multicentre prospective study[6] in combination with other prospective and retrospective data provide excellent reassurance that Mohs surgery as a single treatment modality for incidental, small nerve PNI identified and cleared by the procedure provides the lowest local recurrence rate at 5 years when compared to published data for other treatments. Inclusion in a PNI-specific registry is recommended, with the aim of developing evidence-based treatment algorithms in this subgroup of patients.

New therapies such as cemiplimab and pembrolizumab (monoclonal anti PD-1/PD-L1)—used in locally advanced, inoperable and metastatic SCC—are best managed in the MDT setting, but were not indicated at this stage in this case.

Ongoing close clinical review at two-month intervals for the first two years is recommended and should include complete skin examination, as well as examination of the surgical sites and draining lymph nodes. Concomitant ultrasound examination of cervical lymph nodes achieves higher sensitivity (while avoiding the radiation exposure of repeated CT scans), but with a higher risk of false positives. Education and counselling of patients regarding the risk for recurrence, metastasis and new skin cancers is invaluable to identify issues at an early stage. Ongoing sun protection and regular sunscreen use should be emphasised. Chemoprevention with acitretin and nicotinamide should be considered, although there is limited evidence of benefit.

References

1. Soleymani T, Brodland DG, Arzeno J, Sharon DJ, Zitelli JA. Clinical outcomes of high-risk cutaneous squamous cell carcinomas treated with Mohs surgery alone: An analysis of local recurrence, regional nodal metastases, progression-free survival, and disease-specific death. J Am Acad Dermatol 2023; 88(1): 109–117.
2. Amin MB, Edge SB, Greene FL, Byrd DR, Brookland RK, Washington MK, et al. (eds). AJCC Cancer Staging Manual (8th edition). New York: Springer; 2017.
3. Karia PS, Jambusaria-Pahlajani A, Harrington DP, Murphy GF, Qureshi AA, Schmults CD. Evaluation of American Joint Committee on Cancer, International Union Against Cancer, and Brigham and Women's Hospital tumor staging for cutaneous squamous cell carcinoma. J Clin Oncol 2014; 32(4): 327–334.
4. Ruiz ES, Karia PS, Besaw R, Schmults CD. Performance of the American Joint Committee on Cancer Staging Manual, 8th Edition vs the Brigham and Women's Hospital Tumor Classification System for Cutaneous Squamous Cell Carcinoma. JAMA Dermatol 2019; 155(7): 819–825.
5. Thompson AK, Kelley BF, Prokop LJ, Murad MH, Baum CL. Risk factors for cutaneous squamous cell carcinoma recurrence, metastasis, and disease-specific death: A systematic review and meta-analysis. JAMA Dermatol 2016; 152(4): 419–428.
6. Tschetter AJ, Campoli MR, Zitelli JA, Brodland DG. Long-term clinical outcomes of patients with invasive cutaneous squamous cell carcinoma treated with Mohs micrographic surgery: A 5-year, multicenter, prospective cohort study. J Am Acad Dermatol 2020; 82(1): 139–148.